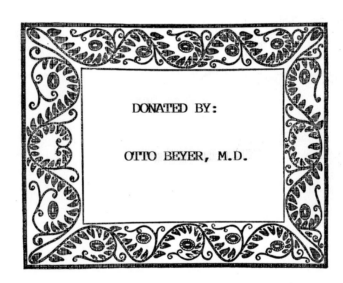

URETEROSCOPY

JEFFRY L. HUFFMAN, M.D.
Assistant Professor of Surgery
Division of Urology
University of Southern California School of Medicine

DEMETRIUS H. BAGLEY, M.D.
Associate Professor of Urology and Radiology
Jefferson Medical College of Thomas Jefferson University

EDWARD S. LYON, M.D.
Professor of Urology and Chief of Endoscopy
Pritzker School of Medicine
University of Chicago

With Contributions By

R. ERNEST SOSA, M.D.
Assistant Professor of Surgery/Urology
James Buchanan Brady Foundation
The New York Hospital
Cornell Medical Center

1988
W. B. SAUNDERS COMPANY
Harcourt Brace Jovanovich, Inc.
Philadelphia • London • Toronto • Montreal • Sydney • Tokyo

W. B. SAUNDERS COMPANY
Harcourt Brace Jovanovich, Inc.

210 West Washington Square
Philadelphia, PA 19105

Library of Congress Cataloging-in-Publication Data

Huffman, Jeffry L.

Ureteropyeloscopy.

Includes index.

1. Ureters-Diseases—Diagnosis.   2. Kidneys-Diseases—Diagnosis.   3. Endoscope and endoscopy.   4. Endoscopic surgery.   I. Bagley, Demetrius H.   II. Lyons, Edward
S.   III. Title.   [DNLM: 1. Endoscopy—methods.
2. Ureteral Diseases—diagnosis.   3. Ureteral Diseases—
therapy. WJ 400 H889u]

RD578.H84   1988   616.6′107545   87–12797

ISBN 0–7216–2148–1

Editor: William Lamsback
Designer: Karen O'Keefe
Production Manager: Peter Faber
Manuscript Editor: Susan Short
Illustrations & Cover by: Philip Ashley
Illustration Coordinator: Walt Verbitski
Indexer: Angela Holt

Ureteroscopy   ISBN   0–7216–2148–1

Last digit is the print number: 9   8   7   6   5   4   3   2   1

Preface

Transurethral endoscopy of the upper urinary tract has rapidly become accepted as a standard urologic procedure. Three major factors have been responsible for making this possible. These are (1) the recognition of the need for and possibility of dilating the ureterovesical junction, (2) the use of techniques for fragmenting large ureteral calculi, and (3) the development of reliable, useful endoscopes. Along with this expanded use of ureteroscopy has come a need for a text that can discuss instruments, indications, and techniques in a manner appropriate for the novice as well as for the intermediate or experienced ureteroscopist.

In this book, we have attempted to discuss the techniques for ureteroscopy in sufficient detail so that the readers can become familiar with the present state of the art and can appreciate some of the pitfalls that have been encountered in its development. Step by step techniques have been described where possible. Basic guidelines for safety factors have been stressed.

Not every instrument or every technique will remain current, yet the state of the art is now on a plateau at which many of the basic guidelines will remain applicable. Instrument development continues with refinement of the basic diagnostic and working endoscopes. Smaller instruments with larger channels and more versatile features will continue to become available. The working instruments and lithotriptors also continue to be refined, yet the basic designs, purposes and limitations remain.

The chapters on passing the ureteroscope and lithotripsy are widely applicable today, and these techniques constitute the major use of endoscopes. As experience accumulates and new instruments develop, the indications for ureteropyeloscopy will continue to grow within the broad outlines discussed. The potential role for ureteroscopy in diagnosing and possibly for treating tumors of the upper urinary tract is overwhelming. The problems and successes encountered in the studies to date constitute the basis for these techniques and will certainly be examined and the indications clarified in the next few years.

Flexible ureteropyeloscopy has grown from an occasional procedure performed when all other endoscopic techniques failed to a major portion of upper tract endoscopy. Flexible endoscopes will undoubtedly continue to play a much greater role in endoscopy within the ureter and intrarenal collecting system.

The complications of ureteropyeloscopy have been few and generally mild, yet individual episodes can be severe. Recognition of these complications and appropriate countermeasures to avoid them can minimize problems in practice. The appendix presents specific difficulties that may arise in the use of ureteroscopes and outlines both the source of the problems and the potential solutions.

Ureteroscopy provides a ready resource for the techniques and results of ureteroscopic procedures and can serve as a focal point for the future development of ureteroscopy. These techniques and instruments have opened the last remaining segment of the urinary tract to endoscopic inspection and manipulation. Every urologist can become familiar with these procedures and add them to his or her repertoire.

Jeffry L. Huffman
Demetius H. Bagley
Edward S. Lyon

Contents

CHAPTER 1

The Development of Instrumentation for Transurethral Ureteropyeloscopy

JEFFRY L. HUFFMAN
DEMETRIUS H. BAGLEY

Instrumentation for transurethral endoscopy of the upper urinary tract has certainly made great strides since Hugh Hampton Young first reported visualizing the ureter and renal pelvis of a young child with a rigid pediatric cystoscope.[1] He was able to pass his instrument to the renal pelvis of a 2-week-old child with massively dilated upper collecting systems secondary to posterior urethral valves, visualizing the interior of the ureter, the renal pelvis, and the renal calyces.

Probably the greatest achievements in the development of instrumentation for the upper urinary tract were by Harold H. Hopkins. One important contribution was the development of the fiberoptic technology that led to flexible fiberoptic endoscopes and enhanced illumination of rigid endoscopes. Another achievement, the invention of the rigid rod lens system, revolutionized light transmission and visualization through rigid endoscopes.

Although the phenomenon of transmission of light through glass fibers had been known since the 1920's,[2, 3] it was not until 1954 that Hopkins and Kapany[4] and van Heel[5] introduced fiberoptics. This led to the development of useful light- and image-transmitting medical instruments, the fiberscopes, and finally the real advantages of fiberoptics in medicine were realized.[6] In 1958, Hirschowitz[7] reported the clinical use of a gastroscope that allowed him to visualize a duodenal ulcer through a completely flexible instrument composed of a light-conducting bundle and an image-transmitting bundle of glass fibers. For coherent image transmission, the fibers in this instrument were spatially arranged exactly the same at the proximal and distal ends of the bundle.

The Flexible Ureteropyeloscopes

Marshall, in 1964,[8] reported using a 3-mm. fiberscope, or ureteroscope, that was passed transurethrally through a 26 F cystoscope and then into the distal ureter, where a ureteral stone was visualized at 9 cm. Although there was excellent transmission of light and images with this flexible ureteroscope, there was no method for changing the direction of the tip of the instrument and no method for irrigation to provide a clear field and adequate distension of the ureter. The small size of this instrument, a necessity for passage through the ureter, prevented the incorporation of a deflecting mechanism and a channel for introducing irrigation fluid with the light- and image-transmitting bundles. This size problem remains a limiting factor today.

Takagi and co-workers began working with a narrow, flexible fiberoptic endoscope in 1966; it was 2.7 mm. in diameter and 70 cm. in length.[9, 10] They reported its use in a patient undergoing an open operation in which the instrument was passed through a ureterotomy to visualize and photograph the renal pelvis and papilla. Once again, the difficulties of not having an irrigating system and of not being able to change the direction of the tip of the instrument were encountered. However, it became evident that it was possible to visualize portions of the urinary tract that could not be viewed through rigid cystoscopes.

Bush and co-workers had also begun working with flexible instrumentation in the late 1960's.[11] Their instrument, inserted cystoscopically like a ureteral catheter, enabled visualization of the upper urinary tract. Irrigation was provided by means of a forced diuresis, and any manipulation was performed with accessories passed alongside the ureteroscope.

The successful use of a pyeloureteroscope passed transurethrally in 23 patients was reported by Takagi and co-workers in 1971.[10] This instrument, an Olympus Model KF, was 2 mm. in diameter and 75 cm. in length. The addition of a 2.5-cm. angulating section at the distal end of the instrument enabled passage of this instrument into the ureteral orifice and through the intramural ureter in the same fashion as a ureteral catheter. It also enabled, with the help of fluoroscopy, passage up the ureter and into major calyces within the renal pelvis. Despite having the advantage of a flexible tip, this instrument still did not have an irrigation system, and as reported by Takagi and co-workers, there were occasional problems with passage of the instrument through the intramural ureter that resulted in breakage of the glass fibers.

To circumvent this problem of pyeloureteroscope insertion, Takayasu and Aso introduced a Teflon guidetube that was passed initially through a special cystoscope with an ocular lens system that protruded at a 45-degree angle from the shaft.[12] The angulation of the lens system helped to prevent fracture of the glass fibers of the instrument as it was pushed through the cystoscope, and a special deflecting bridge limited sharp angulation of the instrument as it passed from the end of the cystoscope. The guidetube was passed into the bladder and engaged by the deflecting bridge. A ureteral catheter was then passed through the guidetube and into the ureteral orifice. Once the catheter was approximately 10 cm. within the ureter, the guidetube was pushed over it in a coaxial fashion. The ureteral catheter could then be removed and replaced with the flexible pyeloureteroscope. Takagi and Aso reported a 100 per cent success rate in 19 patients with this guidetube method compared with an 80 per cent success rate in 50 patients prior to its use. However, once again, the only irrigation system was provided by irrigating through the guidetube or by inducing a diuresis. Therefore, observation of the upper urinary tract was sometimes difficult or impossible in the presence of debris or hematuria.

The Development of Rigid Ureteroscopes

Although first achieved by Young in 1912, rigid ureteroscopy was not performed in a routine fashion until 1977 when Goodman[13] and Lyon and co-workers[14] independently demonstrated the feasibility of deliberate excursions into the ureter. Again it was a contribution of Hopkins that made this possible. His invention of the rigid rod lens system enabled extremely effective light transmission through rigid endoscopes. Using his principles, it was possible to construct instruments small enough to use in the ureter that still provided enough light for effective endoscopy.

The traditional rigid endoscopes prior to this time were constructed of a field lens system that consisted of a tube of air with thin lenses of glass. There were objective lenses at the distal tip of the endoscope and a succession of thin relay lenses refracting the rays of light through the instrument to the eyepiece where they were magnified for the observer.

In 1960, Hopkins invented the rod lens system for rigid endoscopes that is used currently.[15] This system relays the image by a succession of rod lenses separated by air. The thin spaces of air serve as lenses, and the glass serves as space. The effect of this is twofold: (1) the total light transmitted is increased because of the higher refractive index of glass, and (2) rod lenses are easier to mount than thin lenses and a greater diameter lens can be installed for a given diameter endoscope sheath, thus increasing light transmission.

Another factor improving light transmission through the rod lens endoscopes is the use of an efficient multilayer antireflection coating on the surfaces of the lens. All these factors added together provide the modern rod lens endoscope with a total light transmission of approximately 80 times greater than that of the traditional endoscope.

The Rigid Ureteroscopes

Lyon and co-workers' and Goodman's procedures in 1977 were performed initially with pediatric cystoscopes that were 9.5 F in size (Fig. 1–1).

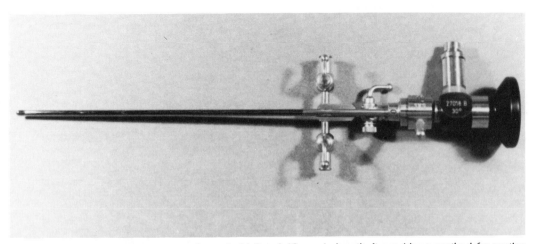

Figure 1–1. The pediatric cystoscope shown is 11 F and 18 cm. in length. It provides a method for routine examination of the distal ureter in women.

Although length was a limiting factor, these instruments could be used to examine the distal ureter and intramural tunnel in female patients and some male patients.

In conjunction with Lyon and co-workers, Richard Wolf Instruments designed an instrument modelled after a juvenile cystoscope, which was specifically used for ureteroscopy (Fig. 1–2).[17] This instrument had a working length of 23 cm. and could readily reach the distal ureter in male and female patients. There were several different rigid sheaths: 13.0, 14.5, and 16.0 F with a 16.0 F resectoscope sheath. The 13.0 F instrument could only be used for observation. A total of 57 procedures were performed with these instruments between 1978 and 1981 with a success rate of 90 per cent.[18] For the first time calculi were visualized directly in the ureter, engaged in a basket under vision, and removed.[19, 20]

This instrument was occasionally very difficult to pass into the ureteral orifice.[21] Its beak was constructed without much bevel, and in order to pass the instrument into the orifice, the trigone had to be depressed while at the same time the instrument was advanced. This often resulted in a blind spot during insertion that prohibited visualization of the ureteral lumen. Not only was insertion difficult and time consuming, but also it was often impossible. False passages occasionally resulted because of this blind spot and subsequent improper alignment of the instrument.[18]

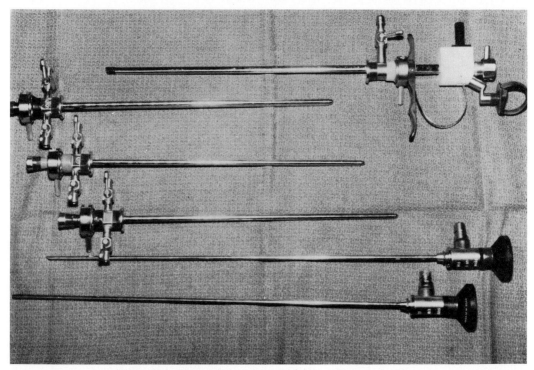

Figure 1–2. The original ureteroscopes used by Lyon were 23 cm. long and had sheath sizes of 13 F, 14.5 F, and 16 F with interchangeable 0 and 70 degree telescopes. The 13 F sheath was for observation only, whereas the 14.5 and 16 F sizes permitted passage of ancillary catheters up to 5 F in size. A 16 F resectoscope sheath (top) with working element was also used.

The Rigid Ureteropyeloscopes

Karl Storz Instruments in conjunction with Perez-Castro made the next significant contribution to the field of rigid ureteroscopy. They introduced an instrument with a working length of 39 cm. that could reach the renal pelvis in male and female patients after transurethral passage (Fig. 1–3).[22] Often this is called the ureterorenoscope; we prefer to designate this instrument as a ureteropyeloscope since only the ureter and renal pelvis can be effectively examined. These instruments were constructed with stated sheath sizes of 9 and 11 F, and each had a 5 F working channel. In conjunction with the 11 F sheath, interchangeable 0 and 70 degree telescopes with their bridges were available for visualization within the ureter and renal pelvis, respectively. An 11 F resectoscope sheath that had a partially insulated beak with an inverted bevel allowed ureteroscopic resection.

Richard Wolf Instruments developed a similar instrument with a 41-cm. working length in stated sheath sizes of 11.5 and 10.0 F (Fig. 1–4). The larger operating sheath had a 5 F channel for accessories, but the smaller sheath was for observation only. A resectoscope sheath that was 11.5 F with a completely insulated beak was also designed (Fig. 1–5). An additional instrument having an integral 5 degree telescope that is 9.5 F with a 5 F working channel is also available from Wolf.

American Cystoscope Makers, Inc. (ACMI) and Olympus have also developed rigid ureteropyeloscopes. The ACMI designs have two lengths (25 and 45 cm.), both 12.5 F in size. These are passed through a cystoscope sheath which is inserted into the bladder. Olympus also has sheaths available that are 12.5 F and 43 and 54 cm. in length. Both manufacturers have interchangeable telescopes (0 and 70 degrees).

Specialized Endoscopes for Ultrasonic Lithotripsy

A major advancement in the field of ureteropyeloscopy occurred with the introduction of ureteroscopic ultrasonic lithotripsy techniques.[23] These techniques revolutionized the endoscopic approach to upper tract calculi. Essentially, any calculus that can be visualized ureteroscopically is fragmented and removed with the help of the ultrasonic transducer. The original probes were 8 F in size and could only be inserted through a standard sheath after the telescope was removed. The metal probes were long enough to reach through the instrument sheath and were hollow to allow exit of stone fragments and irrigant with suction applied to the proximal handle. An ultrasonic generator provides the energy necessary for fragmentation. This connects to the probe by an accessory cord. The generator has variable intensity settings, and the consistency of the stone being fragmented (e.g., cystine versus uric acid) determines which is most effective.

Ureteroscopic instruments designed specifically for use with ultrasonic lithotripsy probes were introduced soon thereafter. These "offset" or "direct-viewing" telescopes had an angled eyepiece to enable simultaneous intro-duction of the solid metal probe, thus allowing ultrasonic fragmentation to be performed under visual control. Karl Storz Instruments, Richard Wolf

Text continued on page 12

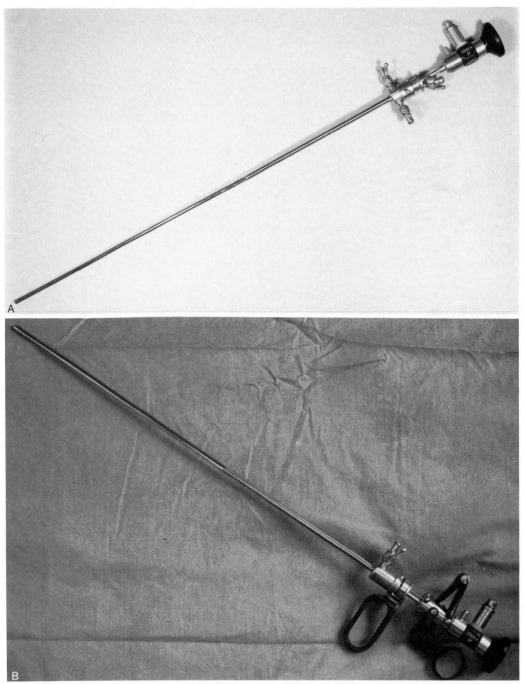

Figure 1–3. A, The original Karl Storz ureteropyeloscope was stated to be 11 F with a working length of 39 cm. There were interchangeable 0 and 70 degree telescopes with their individual bridges. B, The Karl Storz resectoscope is 11 F and has an insulated beak with an inverted bevel for smooth cutting (see Fig. 1–5).

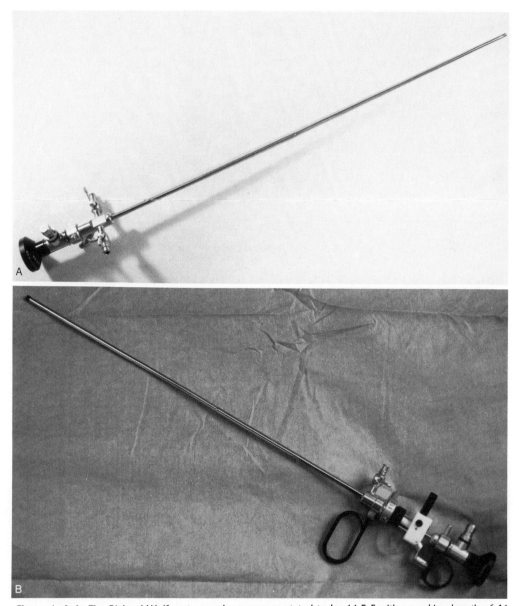

Figure 1–4. A, The Richard Wolf ureteropyeloscope was stated to be 11.5 F with a working length of 41 cm. Interchangeable 5 and 70 degree telescopes were provided; however, they inserted directly into the sheaths without bridges. B, The Richard Wolf 11.5 F resectoscope.

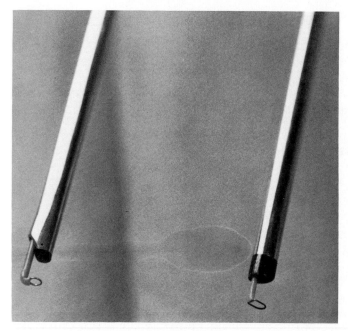

Figure 1–5. The Karl Storz resectoscope loop (Left) and the Richard Wolf loop (Right) have very fine construction to enable excellent control without excessive tissue injury.

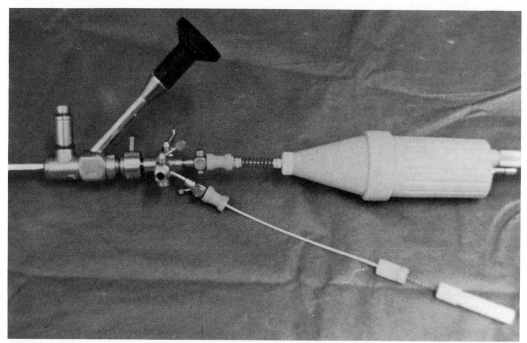

Figure 1–6. The 11.5 F Richard Wolf offset instrument allows simultaneous passage of a 1.5 mm. lithotripsy probe and a 3.5 F stone basket.

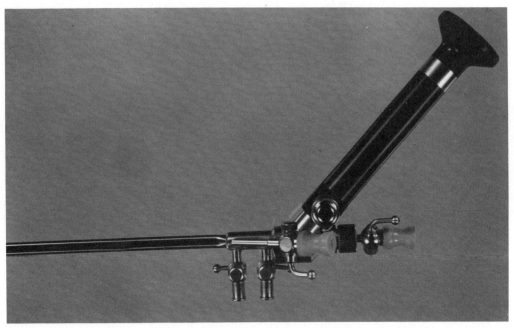

Figure 1–7. The 10.5 F Storz offset ureteroscope has a single working channel for the solid wire ultrasound probe. This endoscope can often be passed into the undilated ureter to fragment even an impacted calculus under direct vision.

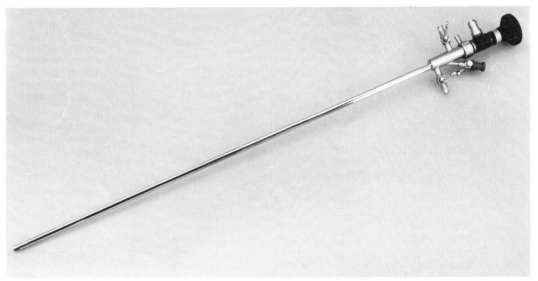

Figure 1–8. This Wolf continuous flow ureteroscope is 12.5 F and has the capacity for interchangeable telescopes and a 5 F working channel for passage of additional accessories.

Instruments, Olympus and ACMI all developed such instruments (Figs. 1–6 and 1–7). Initially, these were constructed with an integral sheath and telescope and had reduced sized probes (1.5 to 2.0 mm.) and a smaller sized catheterizing channel (3.0 to 3.5 F).

Eventually, interchangeable systems were introduced that enabled the standard telescope to be exchanged with the offset telescope. Only one sheath was necessary, and the standard telescope could be used to insert the instrument, which is often very difficult with the angled telescope.[24] Richard Wolf Instruments has designed a system that includes a continuous flow sheath, Albarron deflector and short and long offset operating telescopes (Figs. 1–8 to 1–10). The Karl Storz interchangeable system includes instruments to accept the 1.8 mm. hollow ultrasound probe or the solid wire

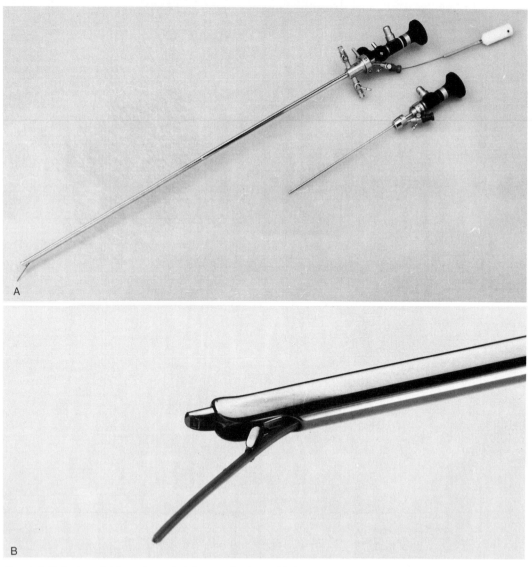

Figure 1–9. A, A pediatric cystoscopic telescope is pictured below a specialized 13.0 F Wolf ureteroscope which accepts a 70 degree lens with an Albarron deflecting lever. B, A close-up view of the distal tip of this instrument shows the Albarron lever deflecting a catheter into the field of view of the 70 degree telescope.

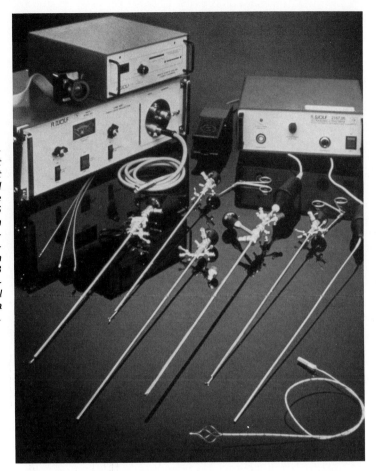

Figure 1–10. The Wolf uretero-scopic system. From left to right are the video camera and cine light source, the cone-shaped metal bougies, the 12.5 F resectoscope with 5 degree lens, the short 11.5 F sheath, the 10.5 F observation sheath, the oblique 12.5 F operating sheath with the 1.5 mm. ultrasonic transducer, the 11.5 F sheath with a 5 F accessory port, the 2.3 mm. ultrasonic transducer. The ultrasonic generator with foot pedal is on top of the cine light, and a 3.5 F basket is at the bottom right.

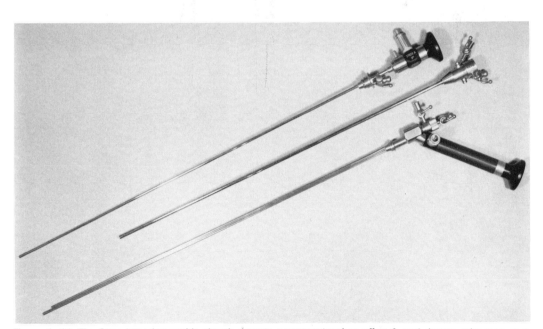

Figure 1–11. The Storz interchangeable sheath accepts a conventional or offset 0 or 6 degree telescope or a lateral viewing telescope. Either the hollow ultrasound probe or the solid wire TUUL (Transurethral Ultrasonic Lithotripsy) probe can be used.

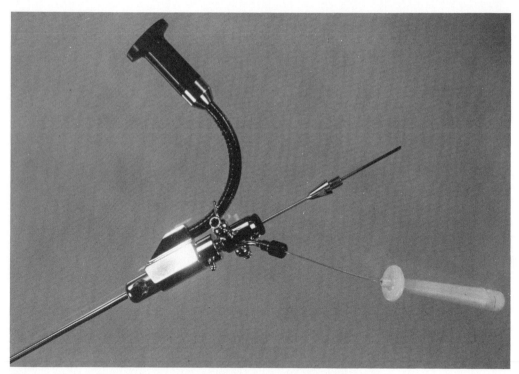

Figure 1–12. *The 12.5 F ACMI operating ureteroscope has a unique "gooseneck" design that permits easier transurethral passage. The simultaneous placement of a stone basket and lithotripsy probe is demonstrated.*

(TUUL) probe (Fig. 1–11). Both long telescopes, which can reach the renal pelvis, and a shorter design, adequate for the lower ureter, are available.

Two companies, ACMI and Olympus, have introduced operating ureteroscopy instruments that combine a rigid sheath with flexible fiberoptic

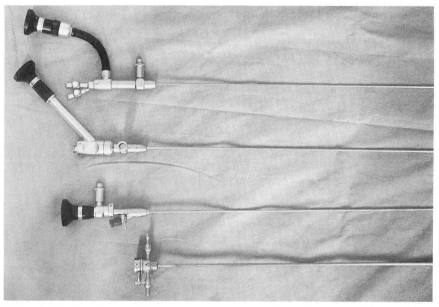

Figure 1–13. *The Olympus rigid ureteroscopes consist of interchangeable (0°) and lateral (70°) lenses, an offset rigid working telescope and an offset flexible fiberoptic telescope (Vari-Flex), which fit into a 10.5 F or a 13 F sheath.*

bundles for illumination and imaging. The eyepiece can be deflected so that it can be positioned conveniently for the urologist's viewing (Figs. 1–12 and 1–13).

References

1. Young HH and McKay RW: Congenital valvular obstruction of the prostatic urethra. Surg Gynecol Obstet 48:509, 1929.
2. Baird JL, British patent 285,738; February 15, 1928.
3. Hansell CW, US patent 1,751,584;1930.
4. Hopkins HH and Kapany NS: A flexible fiberscope, using static scanning. Nature 173:39, 1954.
5. van Heel ACS: A new method of transporting optical images without aberrations. Nature 173:39, 1954.
6. Curtiss LE, Hirschowitz BI, and Peters CW: A long fiberscope for internal medical examination. J Opt Soc Am 46:1030, 1956.
7. Hirschowitz BI, Curtiss LE, Peters CW, and Pollard HM: Demonstration of a new gastroscope, the "fiberscope." Gastroenterology 35:50, 1958.
8. Marshall VF: Fiberoptics in urology. J Urol 91:110, 1964.
9. Takagi T, Go T, Takayasu H, and Hioki R: Small caliber fiberscope for visualization of the urinary tract, biliary tract, and spinal canal. Surgery 64:1033, 1968.
10. Takagi T, Go T, Takayasu H, and Aso Y: Fiberoptic pyeloureteroscope. Surgery 70:661, 1971.
11. Bush IM, Goldberg E, Javadpour N, Chakrobortty H, and Morelli F: Ureteroscopy and renoscopy: a preliminary report. Chicago Med School Q 30:46, 1970.
12. Takayasu H and Aso Y: Recent development for pyeloureteroscopy: guide tube method for its introduction into the ureter. J Urol 112:176, 1974.
13. Goodman TM: Ureteroscopy with pediatric cystoscope in adults. Urology 9:394, 1977.
14. Lyon ES, Kyker JS, and Schoenberg HW: Transurethral ureteroscopy in women: a real addition to the urologic armamentarium. J Urol 119:35, 1978.
15. Hopkins HH, British patent 954,629, and US patent 3,257,902; 1960.
16. Hopkins HH: The modern urological endoscope. In Gow JG and Hopkins HH (eds.): A Handbook of Urological Endoscopy. Edinburgh, Churchill Livingstone, 1978, p. 29.
17. Lyon ES, Banno JJ, and Schoenberg HW: Transurethral ureteroscopy in men using juvenile cystoscopy equipment. J Urol 122:152, 1979.
18. Huffman JL, Bagley DH, and Lyon ES: Extending cystoscopic techniques into the ureter and renal pelvis—Experience with ureteroscopy and pyeloscopy. JAMA 250:2004, 1983.
19. Huffman JL, Bagley DH, and Lyon ES: Treatment of distal ureteral calculi using a rigid ureteroscope. Urology 20:574, 1982.
20. Das S: Transurethral ureteroscopy and stone manipulation under direct vision. J Urol 125:112, 1981.
21. Huffman JL, Bagley DH, and Lyon ES: Transurethral ureteropyeloscopy. In Urologic Endoscopy: A Manual and Atlas. Boston, Little, Brown and Company, 1985, pp. 185–204.
22. Perez-Castro Ellendt E and Martinez-Pineiro JA: Transurethral ureteroscopy—a current urological procedure. Arch Esp Urol 33:445, 1980.
23. Huffman JL, Bagley DH, Schoenberg HW, and Lyon ES: Transurethral removal of large ureteral and renal pelvic calculi using ureteroscopic ultrasonic lithotripsy. J Urol 130:31, 1983.
24. Huffman JL and Clayman RV: Endoscopic visualization of the supravesical urinary tract: transurethral ureteropyeloscopy and percutaneous nephroscopy. Semin Urol 3:60, 1985.

CHAPTER 2

Indications for Ureteropyeloscopy

DEMETRIUS H. BAGLEY

The indications for ureteropyeloscopy have expanded because of the increasingly successful experience with the techniques and the development of newer instruments capable of a wider range of intricate procedures. Just as the earliest attempts at extraction of calculi were limited to the distal ureter in females because of the short pediatric instruments employed, so are the present day limitations of rigid instrumentation and straight, rigid ultrasound techniques for calculus fragmentation probably only temporary limitations. If these barriers can be surpassed, then the indications for ureteropyeloscopic stone removal may no longer be limited to ureteral calculi and occasional renal pelvic calculi. Similarly, additional techniques for the biopsy and treatment of tumors throughout the intrarenal collecting system will expand the indications for ureteropyeloscopic treatment of upper tract urothelial tumors.

Ureteropyeloscopy is generally performed in addition to other standard diagnostic procedures when these techniques fail. It is also used to replace standard therapeutic procedures when an endoscopic technique offers an obvious advantage.

The indications for ureteropyeloscopy can be grouped into several large categories by the disease processes being treated. These include procedures for calculi, foreign bodies, fistulas, obstructions, and tumors. Within each broad group, there are indications for both diagnosis and treatment.

Calculi

The most frequent indication for ureteropyeloscopy is the presence or suspicion of urinary calculi. These techniques are useful for both the diagnosis and treatment of calculi.

DIAGNOSIS

The diagnosis of renal calculi is usually made on the basis of radiographic findings. Often a radiopaque calculus is located within the urinary collecting system, with or without obstruction on excretory urography. In many patients, there may be a suspicion of urinary calculus because of hematuria, pain, a small area of calcification on radiographic films, or a radiolucent lesion. In these patients the diagnosis of calculus and the differentiation of

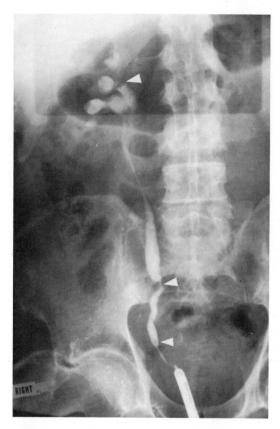

Figure 2–1. In this 63-year-old man who presented with hematuria and right flank pain, an excretory urogram demonstrates a relatively lucent calculus in the distal ureter, a narrow segment at the level of the iliac vessels, and a filling defect in the upper pole infundibulum (arrows). The distal ureteral calculus was retrieved with the conventional ureteroscope, which also allowed diagnosis of the narrow area as edema surrounding a calculus. This calculus was removed by ultrasonic lithotripsy through a direct vision operating ureteroscope. The filling defect could be visualized only with a flexible ureteroscope and was found to be a urothelial tumor.

a filling defect from a urothelial tumor can be made by direct inspection of the lesion and subsequent appropriate treatment (Fig. 2–1).

CALCULUS REMOVAL

The major therapeutic indication for ureteropyeloscopy is the removal of urinary calculi. The indications for calculus removal by the endoscopic approach are the same as those employed for either standard cystoscopic stone manipulation or open surgical removal. The indications, therefore, include severe continued pain, ureteral obstruction, growth of the calculus, failure of the calculus to progress toward the ureteral meatus, and infection (Table 2–1). In each instance the decision regarding active intervention should reflect the patient's desires and the social effects of his stone disease. Calculi located throughout the ureter or even in the renal pelvis may be

Table 2–1
INDICATIONS FOR REMOVAL OF URETERAL CALCULI

Severe Pain	Lack of Progression
Obstruction	Infection
Growth of Calculus	Social Factors

amenable to ureteropyeloscopic removal. The size of the calculus is not a deterrent to ureteropyeloscopic removal now that techniques of ultrasonic or electrohydraulic fragmentation are available (Fig. 2–2).

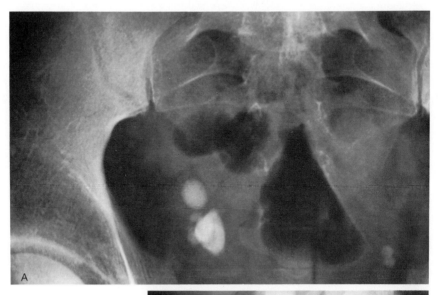

Figure 2–2. A and B, Four large calculi are located in the distal portion of both arms of a duplicated ureter. They were visualized ureteroscopically and removed by ultrasonic fragmentation.

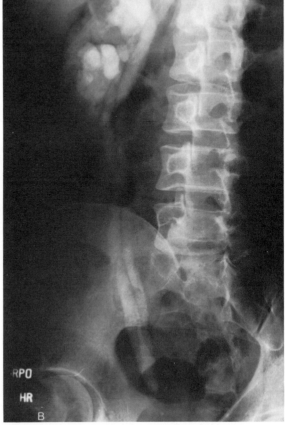

STEINSTRASSE

The fragments of calculi formed from extracorporeal shock wave lithotripsy (ESWL) may fill a portion of the ureter, causing partial or severe obstruction (Fig. 2–3). The need for treatment should be guided by the standard indications for intervention, since such fragment accumulations or steinstrasse, which can be thought of as "logjams," usually pass with minimal symptoms. Although the obstruction can be relieved and the accumulation disrupted by passing a ureter catheter, ureteropyeloscopy is a reliable method of removing the debris. The direct viewing offset lens or operative ureteropyeloscope is particularly useful for fragmenting and removing the calculous debris. The obstructing fragment and the smaller sand-like particles can be broken further and aspirated through the ultrasound probe under vision.

LOCATION OF CALCULUS

The chance of successful stone removal varies with the location of a calculus within the ureter. Although success rates over 90 per cent are observed for distal ureteral calculi, this rate drops to approximately 60 per cent for upper ureteral calculi (see Chapter 7) (Fig. 2–4). Percutaneous techniques and extracorporeal shock wave lithotripsy may be more effective

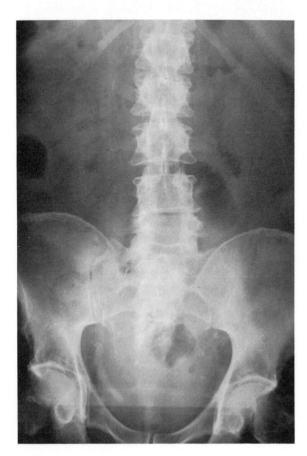

Figure 2–3. A large steinstrasse formed after ESWL from a renal pelvic calculus resulted in severe symptomatic obstruction. The stone fragments were removed with ultrasonic lithotripsy through the direct viewing operating ureteropyeloscope.

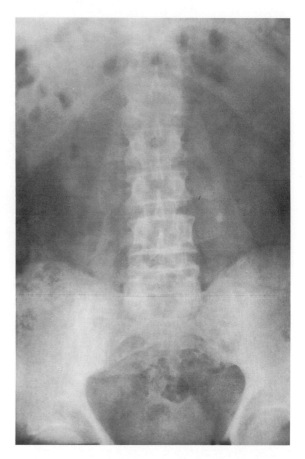

Figure 2–4. This midureteral calculus was removed ureteroscopically. Adequate dilation of the ureter and tilting of the operative table assist in these procedures.

with renal and upper ureteral calculi. However, ureteropyeloscopy can successfully remove upper ureteral calculi primarily or may be helpful in pushing them into the renal pelvis for ESWL. Although distal ureteral calculi can be removed percutaneously, the success rate does not match that achieved with ureteropyeloscopy. ESWL cannot be used for distal ureteral calculi because of the overlapping bony structures. Therefore, in deciding upon an endoscopic or surgical approach for removal of a urinary calculus, the location of the stone and the possibility of successful treatment must be considered as an indication for or against that particular procedure. Uretero-pyeloscopic removal should be considered the treatment of choice for distal ureteral calculi.

Foreign Bodies

The presence or the suspicion of the presence of a foreign body in the ureter or renal pelvis constitutes another major indication for ureteropyelos-copy. Intraluminal foreign bodies can be inspected directly with the uretero-pyeloscope and removed if necessary.

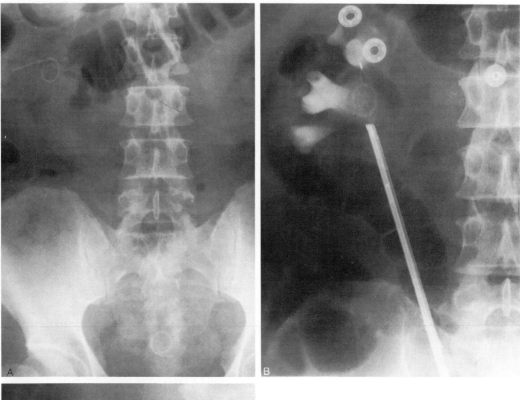

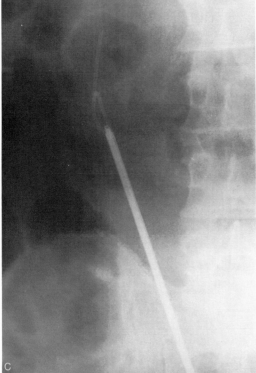

Figure 2–5. A, A 55-year-old patient who had previously had a double pigtail ureteral stent placed for partial right ureteropelvic junction obstruction and had been lost to follow up for two years. On his return, a radiograph of the abdomen revealed a fracture of the indwelling stent with fragments in the kidney and in the bladder. B and C, The ureteropyeloscope was placed to the level of the renal pelvis, and a stone basket was placed around the stent for removal.

DIAGNOSIS

A foreign body within the lumen of the upper tract can usually be diagnosed radiographically or on historical grounds (Fig. 2–5). However, in some rare cases, the exact location may be uncertain. This is more common with radiolucent or slightly radiopaque material. Because of the very limited space within the lumen of the upper urinary tract, any foreign body present can usually be visualized endoscopically. The major difficulty encountered in such examination is usually mucosal edema. Although individuals react differently to different materials, some may have a severe edematous reaction of the mucosa, which obscures the lumen and the foreign body.

REMOVAL

Foreign bodies can be removed endoscopically. Once the structure has been located endoscopically, it can be grasped with a working instrument and removed through the ureteral lumen. The three-pronged grasper, particularly one with a heavy-duty, sharp, pointed design, is valuable for removing foreign bodies. It is often the only instrument that can grasp objects, such as a migrated double pigtail catheter located entirely within the ureter, and hold them firmly enough for removal through the lumen. Small foreign bodies, such as the tip of a stone basket or a portion of a guidewire may be held by a three-pronged grasper or secured with a stone basket or forceps.

Ureteral Obstruction

Ureteropyeloscopy provides a valuable new technique for the diagnosis of, and in some cases the treatment of, ureteral obstruction. Diagnosis is no longer limited to radiologic studies and blind, remote biopsy techniques, now that direct inspection is possible. Similarly, efforts to treat or bypass obstructing lesions can be undertaken with visual monitoring at the site of obstruction rather than by attempting manipulation cystoscopically from the level of the bladder.

Determining the etiology of ureteral obstruction is frequently a diagnostic dilemma. Even the differentiation of extrinsic from intrinsic obstruction, although often suggested by radiologic findings, is frequently uncertain. Direct endoscopic inspection can usually make this distinction (see Figs. 2–1 and 2–6).

Intrinsic obstructive ureteral lesions may be even more difficult to distinguish. The major intrinsic causes of ureteral obstruction include post-inflammatory strictures, urothelial neoplasm, and calculus. Suggestive but not specific indications regarding the nature of intrinsic obstructive ureteral lesions can be gained from the patient's history and the radiologic findings. Benign post-inflammatory strictures may be suspected with a previous history of a calculus, catheterization, tuberculosis, or retroperitoneal disease. The finding on the excretory urogram is usually a regular, narrowed ureteral segment of varying length. No filling defect or calcification is evident. A urothelial neoplasm is often asymptomatic but associated with hematuria.

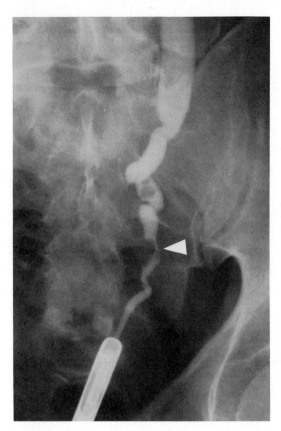

Figure 2–6. *Ureteral obstruction demonstrated on this retrograde pyelogram was the result of a nonurothelial intrinsic neoplasm of the ureter (arrow).*

Radiographically, there may be a filling defect within that segment of the ureter or an irregular outline of the lumen. Urinary cytology often indicates the presence of malignant or atypical cells. Calculi are often associated with some history of pain, usually of sudden onset, and possibly with a previous history of calculi as well. Radiographically, a calcification, even faint or minute, may be present, but radiolucent or very faintly opaque stones may be undetected. Overlying bony structures may obscure calcification. A radiolucent calculus may cause a filling defect on excretory urography to be indistinguishable from that produced by a urothelial neoplasm. In each case, direct endoscopic inspection may indicate the nature of the causative lesion. Although the crystalline structure of a calculus is usually readily apparent, the possibility of calculus formation on a neoplasm cannot be overlooked. It may be more difficult to distinguish a benign ureteral stricture from a urothelial neoplasm; therefore, a biopsy under direct vision with a brush or cup forceps should be done on any lesion that is questionable on inspection alone.

Treatment of obstructive ureteral lesions can often be facilitated endoscopically. Once a diagnosis is made, appropriate therapy can be determined. Even in situations in which a ureteral catheter cannot be passed from the level of the bladder, under direct endoscopic vision a site at which to pass a catheter proximally beyond the obstructing lesion can be located. If identified, other specific lesions can be treated appropriately. A biopsy of a neoplasm can be done, and it may be possible to resect the neoplasm endoscopically. A catheter passed into the proximal urinary system will provide drainage on a temporary basis if open surgical treatment is anticipated. If a calculus is identified, it can usually be removed endoscopically either intact or by fragmentation. A benign stricture can be dilated with a balloon catheter or other instrument, and a stent can be placed to provide adequate drainage during healing.

Fistula

The presence of ureteral fistulas may be an infrequent indication for ureteropyeloscopic intervention. Although most fistulas can be bypassed with a catheter placed by standard cystoscopic techniques, occasionally a catheter cannot be placed from the level of the bladder. It may then be possible to pass the ureteropyeloscope under vision to the site of the fistula, identify the true proximal lumen, and place a catheter to provide proximal drainage and bypass the fistula (Fig. 2–7).

Neoplasm of the Upper Urinary Tract

The presence of an upper urinary tract lesion that is suggestive of neoplasm is another major indication for ureteropyeloscopy. The specific findings indicating the possible presence of a tumor include a filling defect on contrast study, hematuria, abnormal urinary cytology, or previous history of an upper urinary tract filling defect. The endoscopic approach to each of these abnormal entities and the subsequent yield from the study vary.

FILLING DEFECT

The nature of a filling defect noted on radiologic study in the ureter, renal pelvis, or intrarenal collecting system can often be confirmed by visual inspection and biopsy under direct vision. Direct visual inspection can usually distinguish lucent calculi from urothelial neoplasms and possibly distinguish benign ureteral polyps from transitional cell malignancies (Fig. 2–8).

The identification of upper urinary filling defects can be suggested by radiologic studies. Tumors can usually be distinguished from stones by ultrasound or computerized tomographic (CT) scans, since stones demonstrate an acoustic shadow or high density respectively on these studies. However, when the results of these studies are inconclusive or indicate a soft tissue filling defect, then direct visual inspection and biopsy can provide the most accurate diagnosis. Diagnosis can be confirmed by biopsy of the lesion. Brush biopsy under vision affords an accuracy of brushing not possible with radiologic techniques alone. The lesion can be actively brushed under vision, and there will be no question of whether the brush was placed accurately on the lesion. Biopsy of urothelial lesions can also be done directly under vision. A flexible 5 F biopsy forceps fits through the 5 F working

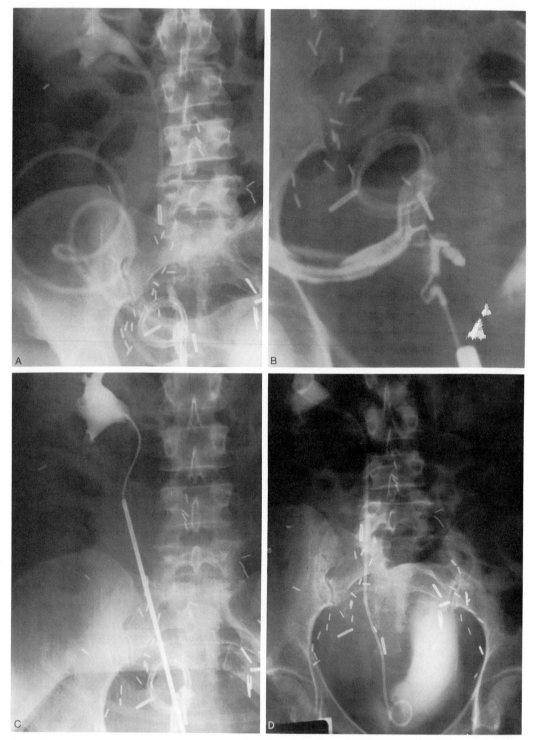

Figure 2–7. A patient who had repair of a ligated ureter developed a persistent uretero-cutaneous fistula demonstrable by excretory urogram (A) and retrograde ureterogram (B). A catheter could not be placed from the level of the bladder. Ureteropyeloscopic inspection revealed the normal ureteral lumen (C) through which a guidewire could be passed for placement of a double pigtail catheter (D). The fistula healed without sequelae.

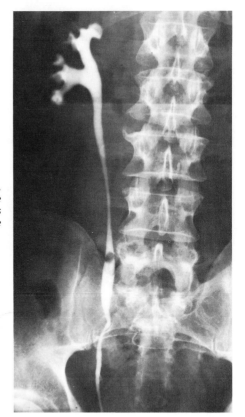

Figure 2–8. This patient, who presented with gross hematuria, was found on excretory urography to have a filling defect in the right mid-ureter. This Grade II transitional cell carcinoma was resected endoscopically without evidence of recurrence for the following two years.

channel of the conventional, sheathed ureteropyeloscope. It can be placed under vision and used to obtain multiple biopsy specimens from the observed lesion. Mapping of the extent of the tumor may also be performed endoscopically in the upper urinary tract just as it is done in the bladder.

An even stronger indication for ureteropyeloscopy in the presence of a urothelial tumor is the potential for treatment of low grade lesions. Limited lesions, particularly in the patient with a solitary kidney, can be destroyed by fulguration with an electrode or even resected. The techniques and early results of such therapy are discussed in Chapter 8.

HEMATURIA

Hematuria is a common presenting symptom of urinary tumors. Thorough evaluation initially includes an excretory urogram and cystoscopy with any appropriate or random biopsies. In a few patients, the source of hematuria can be localized to one or the other ureteral orifice with normal radiologic studies of that collecting system. Direct visual inspection of the upper urinary tract by ureteropyeloscopy is indicated in this select group of patients. The combined use of a rigid ureteropyeloscope for evaluation of the ureter and a flexible instrument for the intrarenal collecting system affords optimal endoscopic surveillance. The rigid instrument offers the best visual resolution in the portion of the collecting system that can be examined, and the flexible instrument offers an extended range and maneuverability for inspection of the intrarenal collecting system (see Chapter 10).

POSITIVE CYTOLOGY

The patient with abnormal urinary cytology indicating transitional cell malignancy, who also has a normal excretory urogram and cystoscopy, including random biopsy specimens, provides another diagnostic dilemma and is a candidate for ureteropyeloscopy. In this situation, the diagnostic accuracy of direct visual inspection and the potential for selected biopsy or selected brushing extend the urologist's diagnostic accuracy. Thus, the indication for ureteropyeloscopy in patients with unilateral positive cytology is very similar to the indication for those with unilateral hematuria. After exhausting standard endoscopic and radiologic studies, ureteropyeloscopy may be used to detect otherwise occult lesions. The value of endoscopic inspection in detecting urothelial lesions not seen radiologically has been demonstrated (see Chapter 8).

PREVIOUS UPPER URINARY MALIGNANCIES

Ureteropyeloscopy also appears to have a role in the surveillance of patients who have previously undergone localized treatment of an upper urothelial malignancy. Whether the lesion has been treated by partial resection or by endoscopic techniques, there remains a risk of local recurrence or the appearance of new primary lesions, and endoscopic surveillance should be continued. Brushing, biopsy, or fulguration of any suspicious or recurrent lesion can then be carried out endoscopically.

Future Indications

The development of new instruments for ureteropyeloscopy may drastically alter the indications for the procedure. At present, the need for ureteral dilation and anesthesia as well as the limited capability for stone fragmentation and tumor destruction are related to the instruments available. The availability of smaller instruments, more flexible instruments, and more effective devices for treating the more common intra-ureteral lesions will undoubtedly expand the indications for ureteropyeloscopy and alter its position in the urologist's armamentarium. As an example, the loss of upper ureteral calculi into the lateral portion of the intrarenal collecting system could almost certainly be overcome if instruments for stone retrieval or fragmentation were available to work with the flexible endoscopes. Similarly, the high success rate for the endoscopic diagnosis of upper urinary tract filling defects could be employed earlier in the evaluation of these patients if a small instrument could be employed in the patient without the need for anesthesia. These instruments are on the horizon and certainly will expand the role of ureteropyeloscopy.

CHAPTER 3

Upper Urinary Tract Anatomy for the Ureteroscopist

JEFFRY L. HUFFMAN
DEMETRIUS H. BAGLEY

A thorough knowledge of the anatomy of the kidney, intrarenal collecting system, and ureter enhances both the safety and success of ureteropyeloscopy. Although anatomic configuration and location of the ureter and renal pelvis vary from one patient to the next, certain endoscopic landmarks remain constant. Similar to the recognition of the bulbous urethra, verumontanum, bladder neck, and trigone in the lower urinary tract, the ureteropyeloscopist must recognize the ureterovesical junction, the pelvic brim, the ureteropelvic junction, and the individual infundibula within the renal pelvis. Just as bronchoscopists recognize and map the bronchi that supply individual lung segments, ureteropyeloscopists should also use similar skill to identify individual major and minor calyces that drain specific regions of renal parenchyma.

Anatomic Relationships of the Kidneys and Intrarenal Collecting System

The right and left kidneys are retroperitoneal organs situated on either side of the vertebral column between the twelfth thoracic vertebra and the third lumbar vertebra (Figs. 3–1 to 3–3). The right kidney is slightly more caudal than the left, with its renal hilus being directly posterior to the descending portion of the duodenum. The right lobe of the liver covers the bulk of its anterior surface and the hepatic flexure of the colon lies directly anterior to the lower pole. The upper pole of the right kidney is in direct contact with the adrenal gland. Immediately anterior to the renal pelvis is the renal vein, which drains into the inferior vena cava medially, and the renal artery. Posteriorly, the kidney is in contact with the psoas, quadratus lumborum, and transversus abdominis muscles from medial to lateral. The diaphragm and the 12th rib overlie the upper pole of the kidney posteriorly.

The left kidney has somewhat different relationships. Posteriorly, the same muscles are encountered as for the right kidney, and the diaphragm and the 12th rib overlie the upper pole. Anteriorly, the tail of the pancreas extends across the renal hilus, and the inferior tip of the spleen covers its anterior border. The proximal jejunum and the splenic flexure of the colon extend across the lower pole of the left kidney anteriorly and the greater curvature of the stomach overlies the left upper pole and adrenal gland.

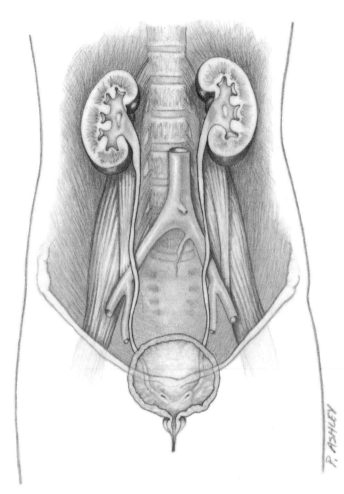

Figure 3–1. *Anteroposterior view of the bladder, ureters, and kidneys. The course of the ureter is noted along the psoas muscle, over the iliac vessels and posteriorly into the bladder.*

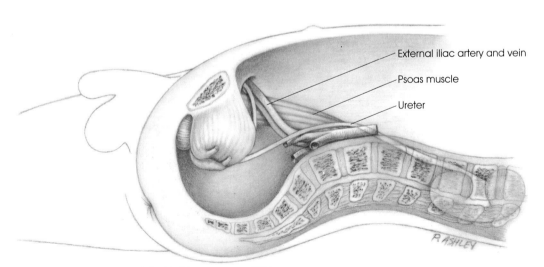

External iliac artery and vein

Psoas muscle

Ureter

Figure 3–2. *Lateral view of the bladder, ureter, and kidney.*

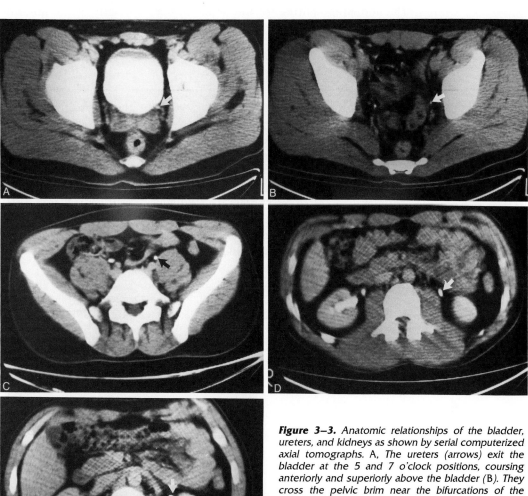

Figure 3–3. Anatomic relationships of the bladder, ureters, and kidneys as shown by serial computerized axial tomographs. A, The ureters (arrows) exit the bladder at the 5 and 7 o'clock positions, coursing anteriorly and superiorly above the bladder (B). They cross the pelvic brim near the bifurcations of the common iliac arteries (C) and continue superiorly immediately anterior to the psoas major muscles (D). The ureters then join the renal pelves, which lie posteriorly at an angle of 70 degrees to the coronal axis of the body (E).

Anatomic Relationships of the Ureters

The ureter is an entirely retroperitoneal structure, extending from the renal pelvis to the bladder (see Figs. 3–1 to 3–3). It varies in length from 28 to 34 cm., with the right being about 1 cm. shorter than the left.

The abdominal portion of the ureter begins superiorly at the uretero-pelvic junction where it is covered by the descending duodenum on the right and the beginning portion of the jejunum on the left. As it courses inferiorly from the renal pelvis, it lies lateral to the inferior vena cava and anterior to the psoas major muscle and the genitofemoral nerve. It then courses slightly medially to cross the ventral surface of the transverse processes of the 3rd to 5th lumbar vertebral bodies and then crosses the bifurcation of the common iliac artery at the hypogastric artery. Near this level, it lies directly posterior to the right colic and ileocolic blood vessels and terminal ileum on the right and the left colic vessels and the line of attachment of the sigmoid mesocolon on the left.

The pelvic portion of the ureter begins as it crosses the bifurcation of the common iliac vessels and enters the true pelvis. As it courses inferiorly, it lies ventral to the hypogastric artery and medial to the obturator nerve and artery. It then runs slightly laterally and posteriorly along the lateral pelvic wall to the region of the ischial spine. At this level, it bends medially and anteriorly to reach the bladder at the ureterovesical junction.

The ureterovesical junction is the narrowest portion of the ureter and corresponds to the entrance of the ureter through the detrusor hiatus in the bladder wall musculature. At this level the ureters are approximately 5.0 cm. apart. As the intramural ureter exits this muscular hiatus, it courses submucosally approximately 2 cm. within the bladder and ends at the ureteral orifice. It is this anatomic configuration of the submucosal ureter that is thought to allow it to preserve its anti-reflux mechanism.

Blood Vessels, Lymphatics, and Nerve Supply of the Ureter and Renal Pelvis

The abdominal ureter and renal pelvis receive their arterial blood supplies from the gonadal and renal arteries and occasionally from capsular or aortic arteries. The lower ureter is supplied by the middle hemorrhoidal and superior vesical arteries, but ureteral arteries may also arise from the common iliac, external iliac, gluteal, deferential, or uterine arteries. When these vessels reach the ureter, they divide into ascending and descending branches located in the tunica adventitia. The venous drainage of the ureter follows the arterial routes.

The ureteral lymphatics begin in the muscle layer and tunica adventitia and drain into regional lymph nodes. In the lower ureter, drainage is to the hypogastric nodes in the pelvis, and in the upper ureter drainage is to the para-aortic or vena caval lumbar nodes.

The sympathetic nerve supply to the ureter is from pre-ganglionic fibers arising in the 11th and 12th thoracic and 1st lumbar spinal segments. The parasympathetic nerve supply to the upper ureter is from the celiac plexus, probably mediated by vagal fibers. Supply to the lower ureter is by way of the 2nd, 3rd, and 4th sacral segments. Afferent fibers from the lower ureter reach the spinal cord (S2, S3, and S4) by means of the pelvic nerve plexus. The upper ureter sends afferents to the 11th and 12th thoracic and 1st lumbar spinal cord segments.

Histologic Structure of the Renal Pelvis and Ureter

The renal pelvis and ureter are thin-walled structures (1 to 2 mm. thick when distended) composed of three layers: fibrous, muscular, and mucosal (Figs. 3–4 and 3–5). The outermost layer is the fibrous layer or tunica adventitia. This is a continuous fibrous structure that runs from the renal sinus along the ureter and inserts into the fibrous coat of the bladder. The most distal aspect of this layer as it inserts into the bladder contains the specialized group of muscle fibers and fibrous tissue known as Waldeyer's sheath. Nerve fibers, lymphatics, and blood vessels are also contained in the tunica adventitia, which is joined externally by adipose tissue surrounding the ureter.

The middle portion is the muscular layer or tunica muscularis. It consists of two poorly defined, thin layers in the renal pelvis and proximal ureter: the inner circular and outer longitudinal. Most often these layers are

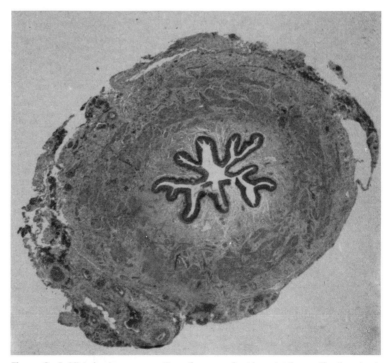

Figure 3–4. Histologic cross-section of a normal mid-ureter (magnification, 1 ×).

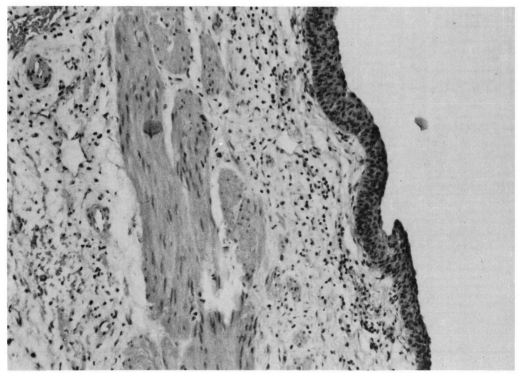

Figure 3–5. *Histologic cross-section of a normal renal pelvis (magnification, 4×).*

indistinct and are found in small bundles running in oblique directions separated by large amounts of connective tissue.

There are three distinct layers in the middle and distal ureter: inner longitudinal, middle circular, and outer longitudinal fibers. The inner longitudinal fibers are more developed near the bladder, and the circular fibers decrease in size at this level.

Within the intramural ureter, the longitudinal muscle fibers also decrease in number and size as the ureteral orifice is approached. In the submucosal ureter there is only a semicircle of longitudinal fibers around the lateral aspect of the ureter, with the medial portion having few muscle fibers at this level. This configuration helps to illustrate why great care must be taken when dilating the tunnel and passing the ureteropyeloscope. Perforation or submucosal false passages occur more easily at this level partly because of the sparse muscular coating.

The innermost lining of the ureter and renal pelvis is the mucosal layer. The anatomic features of this layer give rise to one of the unique properties of the ureter and pelvis: their ability to stretch and distend without rupturing. It consists of epithelium formed by transitional cells and subepithelium (lamina propria) formed by connective tissue.

The epithelium becomes thicker in the distal ureter as compared to that found in the minor calyces. It is approximately two cell layers thick in the calyces and becomes about five or six cell layers thick in the distal ureter near the bladder. The lamina propria contains dense collagenous tissue with many elastic fibers and is continuous with the renal interstitial tissue.

The mucosal layer also contains many longitudinal folds or rugae. These give the non-distended or contracted ureter its characteristic star-shaped appearance when viewed ureteroscopically.

Endoscopic Anatomy of the Intrarenal Collecting System[4]

As urine is drained through the collecting ducts within the renal pyramids, it exits into the minor calyces via the renal papillae. The papillae form the apex of the renal pyramids and vary in number from four to twelve, depending on the individual. Endoscopically, a papilla appears as a rounded cone with a pink, easily friable epithelium. The cupped minor calyx surrounding each papilla is called the calyceal fornix. Occasionally, more than one papilla may project into a minor calyx. These compound calyces occur more commonly in the upper pole.

The four to thirteen minor calyces coalesce at their apices and empty into two or three major calyces, which drain directly into the renal pelvis. Endoscopically, upon entering the renal pelvis from the transureteral route, the bases of the major calyces leading to the upper, middle, and lower poles of the kidney are the first structures visible. They appear as cylindrical openings branching from the pelvis. Often minor calyces are visible in the background. The tubular portion or infundibulum connects the apex to the base of each major calyx.

Separating the major calyces as they branch from the renal pelvis are carinae. Anatomically, these are similar in appearance to the branching of the trachea into the right and left mainstem bronchi. However, there are usually two carinae separating the three major calyceal infundibula.

The endoscopic anatomy of the renal pelvis is extremely variable, with many differences in size, shape, and location. The renal pelvis is considered conical in shape with the apex of the cone representing the ureteropelvic junction. Intrarenal pelves, lying entirely within the renal sinus are small with short infundibula. Extrarenal pelves are usually capacious, lying entirely outside the renal sinus and often having long, narrow infundibula.

The renal pelvis empties urine into the proximal ureter through the ureteropelvic junction. This is one of the naturally narrow portions of the ureter. Endoscopically, it is identified easily as the junction between the relatively narrow ureter and the markedly more capacious renal pelvis. The movement of the pelvis and proximal ureter with each respiratory excursion of the kidney is also readily apparent. Usually a lip of ureteral mucosa is visible within the ureteral lumen near the ureteropelvic junction. As will be discussed in the next section, this anatomic landmark signifies the close proximity of the renal pelvis.

Endoscopic Anatomy of the Ureter

The normal ureter is relatively uniform in caliber and easily distensible; however, there are three naturally occurring, relatively narrow sites within the lumen that are recognizable ureteroscopically: the ureteropelvic junction, the pelvic brim, and the ureterovesical junction. The degree of narrowing that is encountered endoscopically varies from one individual to another. Often the narrowing is not noticeable; however, occasionally the amount of narrowing is such to prohibit passage of the ureteropyeloscope without mechanical dilation.

Besides these anatomic regions, there are other landmarks to be observed. The portion of the ureter as it crosses the termination of the common iliac artery can often be seen pulsating, thus signifying the close approximation of the ureteral and arterial lumens. As discussed previously, the approach of the proximal ureter is signified by its movements with respiration. Each inspiration causes the diaphragm to push downward on the kidney, leading to simultaneous caudal movement of the renal pelvis and proximal ureter. The junction between the fixed and mobile portions of the ureter has a characteristic appearance and signifies the close proximity of the renal pelvis. A bend or lip of mucosa corresponds to this junction. It is located in the posterolateral lumen and is accentuated during inspiration, becoming barely perceptible during expiration.

References

1. Bulger RE: The urinary system. In Weiss L (ed.): Histology—Cell and Tissue Biology. New York, Elsevier Biomedical, 1983, pp. 869–913.
2. Davis JE, Hagedoorn JP, and Bergmann LL: Anatomy and ultrastructure of the ureter. In Bergman H (ed.): The Ureter. New York, Springer-Verlag, 1981, pp. 55–70.
3. Gray H: The urogenital system. In Goss CM (ed.): Anatomy of the Human Body. Philadelphia, Lea & Febiger, 1973, pp. 1265–1339.
4. Huffman JL, Bagley DH, and Lyon ES: Normal anatomy of the ureter and kidney. In Bagley DH, Huffman JL, and Lyon ES (eds.): Urologic Endoscopy. A Manual and Atlas. Boston, Little, Brown and Company, 1985, pp. 13–18.
5. Verlando JT: Histology of the ureter. In Bergman H (ed.): The Ureter. New York, Springer-Verlag, 1981, pp. 13–54.
6. Markee JE: The urogenital system. In Anson BJ (ed.): Morris' Human Anatomy. New York, McGraw-Hill, 1966, pp. 1457–1537.

CHAPTER 4

Preparation for a Ureteroscopic Procedure

JEFFRY L. HUFFMAN
DEMETRIUS H. BAGLEY

Many ingredients contribute to successful completion of a ureteropye-loscopic procedure, and the most important of these is the actual passage of the instrument with stone extraction or tumor biopsy. However, a part of the procedure that is critical to success is proper preoperative planning and thorough discussion with the patient regarding the procedure and the expected results. This is especially critical for a new procedure that is unfamiliar not only to the urologist but also to the patient and operating room staff. Improper preparation, such as (1) not having the necessary ancillary catheters, (2) having instruments that do not function properly, or (3) using an operating room table that cannot be accommodated to the requirements of ureteropyeloscopy, often leads to unsuccessful results.

Preliminary Patient Interview and Preparation

The preoperative patient interview includes: (1) taking a thorough history of prior medical illnesses and surgical procedures, (2) performing a complete physical examination, and (3) obtaining the operative consent from the patient.

As with other surgical and medical procedures, the patient's history is the most valuable part of the evaluation. A thorough history is necessary to establish the indication for any ureteropyeloscopic procedure. As an example, ureteropyeloscopic stone removal has been performed on the basis of indications identical to those used for cystoscopic or open surgical removal of calculi. Prominent among the indications are the patient's desire for relief from the symptoms resulting from the presence of the calculus.

Of major importance is the patient's previous history of surgical procedures. Passage of the ureteropyeloscope to the renal pelvis requires an intact collecting system with a capacious ureter that is mobile and not scarred by previous surgical manipulation. Often a patient's history gives clues that predict problems in instrument passage (Table 4–1). A previous radical prostatectomy (Fig. 4–1) or radical hysterectomy may leave the ureter fixed in the retroperitoneum, and similarly, any ureteral surgery such as uretero-neocystostomy or ureterolithotomy leads to scarring and ureteral immobility. We have found re-implanted ureters to be difficult to dilate; they often require a variety of methods for successful dilation (see Chapter 5). A cross trigonal ureteral re-implant would probably not be accessible endoscopically because of the oblique angle that results with the plane of the posterior

43

Table 4–1
FACTORS IN HISTORY THAT PREDICT DIFFICULT
URETEROPYELOSCOPY

Previous Pelvic Surgery
  Radical Retropubic Prostatectomy
  Total Abdominal Hysterectomy
  Abdominal Perineal Colon Resection
Previous Ureteral Surgery
  Ureterolithotomy
  Ureterolysis
  Ureteroneocystostomy
Obstructive Voiding Symptoms
  Median Lobe Prostatic Hypertrophy
  Urethral Stricture Disease

urethra. Symptoms indicative of bladder outlet obstruction may signify a problem that will make the initial introduction of the ureteropyeloscope difficult. Problems such as urethral stricture, prostatic enlargement, or bladder neck contracture may have to be treated prior to ureteropyeloscopy.

Physical examination of the patient may also give clues that help predict problems (Table 4–2). In both male and female patients a bimanual examination allows assessment of mobility of the urethra, bladder, and lower ureter. Successful ureteropyeloscopy depends on bladder neck and urethral

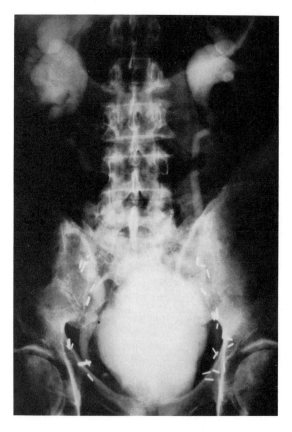

Figure 4–1. This radiograph, taken during an excretory urogram, shows an impacted distal right ureteral calculus in a patient who previously underwent a radical retropubic prostatectomy with bilateral pelvic lymph node dissection. The bladder neck was immobile; however, it was possible to negotiate the distal 3 cm. of the ureter and remove the calculus successfully. It was not possible to pass the ureteroscope any farther proximally.

Table 4–2
FINDINGS ON PHYSICAL EXAMINATION THAT PREDICT
DIFFICULT URETEROPYELOSCOPY

Frozen Pelvis on Bimanual Examination
   Locally Invasive Malignancy
   Diffuse Inflammatory Process
   Previous Radical Surgery or Irradiation
Hypertrophy of the Prostate
Pelvic Mass Displacing the Bladder or Proximal Ureter
Limited Range of Motion of the Hip

mobility. Those that are immobile or frozen may not allow straightening for passage of the rigid instrument.

The patient's general physical appearance may also be important. It may be difficult to pass a ureteropyeloscope into the mid- and proximal ureter in young, muscular males. The combination of a relatively rigid perineal diaphragm and a high psoas muscle can make placement of the instrument difficult.

Benign prostatic hypertrophy may make access into the ureteral orifice impossible. Certainly median lobe hypertrophy, which totally obscures the ureteral orifices, may not allow ureteropyeloscopic entry. Hip mobility also needs to be assessed. Those patients with limited range of motion at the level of the hip may not be candidates for ureteropyeloscopy. Access into the ureter with a rigid instrument depends upon abduction and flexion of the contralateral hip.

It is also necessary to obtain informed consent from the patient preoperatively. Patients should understand that ureteropyeloscopy is a relatively new procedure. Although it has been performed on hundreds of patients throughout the world, there is no long post-operative follow up in most series. Although the goal of the procedure is to prevent an open operation, surgery may still be necessary if the procedure is unsuccessful or if complications arise. Certainly the majority of calculi can be removed ureteropyeloscopically with one procedure. However, the patient should be aware, in advance, that to become stone-free a second ureteroscopy procedure may be necessary, and that a percutaneous nephrostolithotomy, extracorporeal shock wave lithotripsy (ESWL), or open lithotomy may be required. Although relatively few complications have been attributed to ureteropyeloscopy, the patient should be aware of the expected hematuria and of the possibility of infection. The rare occurrence of instrument breakage or late ureteral stricture may also be noted.

Preoperative Examination of Radiographs

Each upper tract collecting system has a slightly different anatomic configuration and relationship to surrounding organs. These differences may be congenital or secondary to pathologic abnormalities, such as obstruction with proximal ureteral dilation and tortuosity. Similar to a motorist's requiring a road map to reach his or her destination by an efficient and safe route, the urologist requires radiographs to successfully reach a "destination" in the upper urinary tract. Usually the studies used to diagnose a lesion for which ureteropyeloscopy is planned are available for the procedure. These radiographs include: excretory urograms with oblique projections, computerized tomograms, and probably the most useful study, a cone-tip retrograde ureteropyelogram. This study provides information regarding ureteral position, tortuosity, and distensibility. If relatively non-distensible portions of the ureter are identified on ureterographs, preparation for the procedure includes securing appropriate instrumentation for upper tract dilation such as dilating balloon catheters, guided olive-shaped bougies, 70-cm. graduated dilators, and a C-arm fluoroscopic unit.

Instrument Preparation

Much of the instrumentation for ureteropyeloscopy is specially designed for the procedure and, in most cases, does not allow substitution. For this reason all instrumentation must be checked prior to initiation of the procedure to ensure its working effectiveness. All endoscopes, working instruments, and stone fragmentation equipment must be available and in good functioning capacity. For instance, an ultrasonic transducer has a limited lifetime after which it does not provide 100 per cent operating capacity. The time to learn of any defects is before the procedure starts.

The appropriate endoscope should be available for the planned procedure. If there is any possibility that a calculus to be removed is too large to pass through even the dilated ureter, then a lithotripter must be available. If an offset operating ureteropyeloscope is to be used for the procedure, then an appropriate-size ureteral ultrasound probe must be available. Confusion may result from the various sizes of ureteral probes available, and the urologist should be certain that the size that will fit through the instrument is available for that procedure. Similarly, the availability of a resectoscope or biopsy forceps should be determined before initiating a ureteropyeloscopic evaluation of a patient with a ureteral filling defect.

The appropriate working instruments should be considered preoperatively (Table 4-3). Stone baskets, ureteral dilators, and a variety of catheters should be in adequate supply. More than one type of ureteral dilator is often needed, and it is advisable to have a set of metal bougies (guided and unguided), a set of 70-cm. graduated dilators, and balloon dilating catheters available for immediate use. A wide assortment of stone baskets is often necessary including 3.0- and 4-F sheaths; 3-, 4-, and 6-wire basket designs; and 8-, 11-, and 15-mm. diameter baskets. Other recommended accessories include: double pigtail stents, single pigtail diversionary stents, three-pronged grasping forceps, biopsy forceps, and grasping snares.

The Operating Room

The operating room used for ureteropyeloscopy should have features that can benefit what may be a long and difficult endoscopic procedure. The specialized ureteropyeloscopic endoscopes and working instruments should

Table 4–3
ACCESSORY INSTRUMENTATION FOR URETEROPYELOSCOPY

Stone Baskets (3.0–5.0 F)
   3-, 4-, and 6-Wire Baskets
   8-, 11-, and 15-mm. Diameter Baskets
Ureteral Dilators
   Metal Conical Bougies
   Guided Metal Bougies (with 0.038-inch guidewire)
   70-cm. Graduated Dilators (with 0.038-inch guidewire)
   Balloon Dilating Catheters
Forceps
   Grasping
   Biopsy
   Three-Pronged Grasping
   Snares
Catheters
   Double Pigtail Stents
   Single Pigtail Diversion Stents
   Open end Catheters
   4- and 5-F Whistle-Tipped Catheters

be readily available to the room. There should be sufficient space to allow use of the appropriate light source, lithotripters, a table that will hold the long rigid endoscopes, and the necessary radiographic equipment.

It is essential to have some radiographic capability. It is most convenient to have a fluoroscopic unit, either a built-in fluoroscope or a portable C-arm image intensifier. Alternatively, an instrument to obtain permanent radiographs is adequate. Optimally, both instruments should be available.

The operating table should have features that permit effective ureteropyeloscopy. It is essential to have a radiolucent table to permit radiographic study during or at the conclusion of the procedure. It is also valuable to be able to change the position of the table in three dimensions: height, head to foot tilt, and lateral tilt. There is also benefit in a table with stirrup supports (Fig. 4–2).

Personnel

Ureteropyeloscopy is not a procedure that can be done by a single person. It is essential to have at least two assistants, one to circulate and one to assist in placing instruments. A scrubbed assistant is necessary because it is virtually impossible for the endoscopist alone to place a long instrument, such as an ultrasonic lithotripter probe, into the ureteropyeloscope and maintain its position at the same time. That same assistant must be familiar with the instruments so that he or she is confident and able to find the appropriate instrument and to anticipate the endoscopist's needs.

Operating Time

The operating time for ureteropyeloscopy can vary widely and depends on several factors. We generally schedule any ureteropyeloscopic procedure

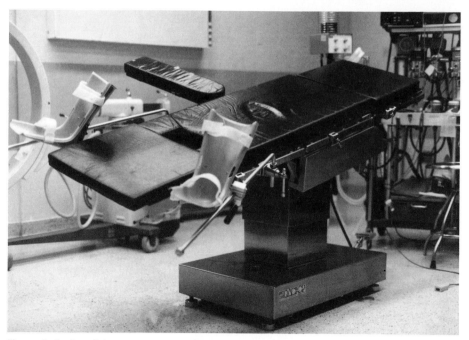

Figure 4–2. A radiolucent operating table that provides two directional tilt as well as height adjustment is a valuable instrument for use during ureteroscopy.

for 2 hours. Although some procedures, particularly the removal of small distal ureteral calculi, may be very short, the other associated procedures, including induction of anesthesia, positioning, preparation, and ureteral dilation, use time in the operating room in addition to the time required for removal of the calculus itself. More complicated procedures such as fragmentation of large calculi or flexible ureteropyeloscopy for evaluation of gross hematuria may require a longer time for the procedure itself in addition to the preparatory steps.

Anesthesia for Transurethral Ureteropyeloscopy

General anesthesia has been recommended for transurethral ureteroscopy and pyeloscopy. There are two reasons that make its use valuable: (1) pain from the ureteral dilation, and (2) movement of the proximal ureter and renal pelvis with each excursion of the diaphragm with respiration. Although spinal or epidural anesthesia is effective to control pain, the respiratory movements of the kidney are not controlled. With the ureteropyeloscope in the upper tract, any coughing or sudden upper body movement could cause inadvertent perforation of the collecting system by the relatively sharp beak of the instrument. General anesthesia with controlled respiration enables the urologist to predict respiratory movement and advance the instrument through the ureteropelvic junction in a safe manner.

Table 4—4
CHECKLIST FOR URETEROPYELOSCOPY

1. History and physical examination
2. Discussion of procedure with patient and informed consent
3. Review of radiographs
4. Necessary catheters, stone baskets, and dilators
5. Instruments functioning well, including ultrasonic generator and probes
6. General anesthesia

Spinal or epidural anesthesia may be suitable for occasional distal ureteral procedures, since this area is not affected by respiratory movements. However, the urologist should be careful to drain the ureter frequently, since distension of the renal pelvis may also induce nausea and vomiting during regional anesthesia. Some urologists have performed ureteropyeloscopy with local anesthesia alone. We have had limited experience with this technique with rigid instruments but have found it useful with the smaller flexible endoscopes. Adequate analgesia could be obtained even for ureteral dilation with significant systemic sedation along with intra-urethral anesthetic.

Summary

In general, for transurethral ureteropyeloscopy, proper preparation and planning increases the chance of success. Thorough preliminary patient evaluation including history, physical examination, and review of radiographic studies helps predict problems in advance and allows the urologist to be equipped to overcome any obstacles. Careful preliminary discussion with the patient regarding the relatively limited experience with the technique, the possibility of complications, and the possibility of an open operation still being necessary is required. Also, all instrumentation that may be required must be secured in advance and checked to ensure that it functions well. See the checklist for ureteropyeloscopy in Table 4—4.

CHAPTER 5

Dilation of the Ureterovesical Junction and Ureter

DEMETRIUS H. BAGLEY

Dilation of the ureterovesical junction including the intramural portion of the ureter is essential for passing most rigid or flexible ureteropyeloscopes. Dilation of the ureter in a controlled fashion minimizes the risk of injury since it provides a lumen adequate for introduction of the instrument and for removal of many calculi.

History

Dilation of the ureter has been employed previously for various indications. Lewis, in 1906,[1] commented on the benefits of dilating the ureterovesical junction to facilitate the passage of ureteral calculi. Others have used the techniques of ureteral dilation to enlarge functionally insignificant but anatomically small ureters in an attempt to relieve flank discomfort and other various maladies. The indications and results were so ill-defined that these techniques have retreated into the historical aspects of urology.

Several techniques and instruments were specifically described in the earlier literature for enlarging the distal ureteral lumen. The use of ureteral catheters is perhaps the simplest technique for dilation. Standard catheters with whistle or other tip configurations of increasing diameter are passed into the ureter cystoscopically. Other catheters, designed with an enlarged segment that has a greater diameter than the main shaft of the catheter, can more effectively dilate the ureter to a larger diameter. The Braasch bulb catheter is an example of these instruments. Multiple catheters can dilate the ureter even more effectively.

Dourmashkin[2] described metal cone-shaped dilators that could be passed into the orifice under direct vision. The tips were interchangeable and could be attached to a flexible carrier handle. The intramural ureter was dilated as large as 20 F if necessary to accommodate the calculus. The same author used rubber bags on catheters to dilate the ureter to facilitate passage of ureteral calculi,[3] and with these instruments he was able to carry the dilation to 24 F if necessary.

Ureteral Dilation for Ureteropyeloscopy

Since the lumen at the normal ureterovesical junction is only approximately 3 mm. in diameter, dilation is essential before passing the rigid

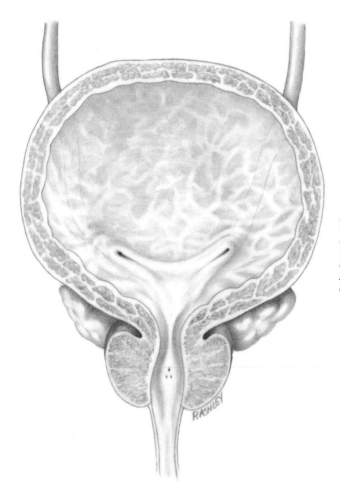

Figure 5–1. The lumen of the intramural ureter is compressed by the muscular bladder wall. The oblique tunnel and the intravesical extension of the ureter provide a one-way flap valve to prevent reflux. The smooth muscle of the ureter itself is mainly oriented in longitudinal bundles at this level.

operating ureteropyeloscopes (Fig. 5–1). Although some of the smaller flexible ureteropyeloscopes can be accepted in the lumen without prior dilation, the lumen must be enlarged for the larger flexible instruments or for introducer sheaths.

The ureter proximal to the bladder is usually adequate to accept a ureteropyeloscope, and dilation is not necessary. The low pressure of the irrigating fluid usually distends the lumen sufficiently for visualization. However, there are frequently segments of ureter that do not distend. These are usually short bands only 2 to 3 mm. in width, but they may be more extensive. A cone-tip retrograde pyelogram is most helpful in delineating the areas that will not distend with irrigation pressure alone. These segments must be dilated prior to passing the ureteropyeloscope.

Several different techniques have provided adequate dilation of the intraluminal ureter. The lumen can be enlarged by placing a ureteral catheter or stent cystoscopically and leaving it in place for one or more days. Greater dilation can be obtained by placing multiple or successively larger ureteral catheters over a period of several days. Acute dilation can be performed with unguided metal cone-shaped bougies or with standard bulb-tipped ureteral catheters.[4] Other dilators are designed to be passed over a guidewire within the ureter. These include graduated dilators similar to Amplatz fascial dilators, balloon catheters, and olive-tipped metal dilators. Others workers have reported success with a system of telescoping or coaxial Teflon dilators.[5]

Subacute or Chronic Techniques for Ureteral Dilation

URETERAL CATHETER

A ureteral catheter placed within the lumen of the ureter will, over one to several days, cause ureteral dilation. One of the early descriptions of ureteropyeloscopy advocated ureteral catheter dilation.[6] By that author's technique, a ureteral catheter is passed cystoscopically into the ureter to be dilated and left in place for 24 hours. At the end of that period, the ureter is sufficiently dilated to permit insertion of the rigid ureteropyeloscope without further enlargement. Others have advocated a several-day period of catheterization before adequate dilation is achieved.

A ureteral catheter of essentially any tip configuration (whistle, olive, or corkscrew) can be passed into the ureter to the level of the renal pelvis. If there is a calculus present, the catheter then drains the proximal portion of the urinary tract. The largest catheter that will easily fit into the ureter is passed endoscopically by standard techniques. Multiple catheters may be placed to dilate the ureter further (Fig. 5–2). The ureteral catheter is secured in position by placing a Foley catheter into the bladder and tying the two catheters together, attaching each to a drainage bag. After the selected period, the ureter will be sufficiently dilated to accept the ureteropyeloscope.

This procedure for dilation is usually easy to perform, since standard techniques of ureteral catheterization are employed. It may be difficult to pass an obstructing calculus. Catheters can be used to dilate the entire ureter and have the advantage of providing urinary drainage.

The major disadvantages of this technique are the time required for full dilation and the mucosal inflammation that develops as a result of the presence of foreign bodies within the ureter and the bladder. Catheter dilation should not be used when ureteropyeloscopy is being performed to evaluate a filling defect, since the catheter may damage or remove a urothelial lesion and thus hinder the diagnostic procedure.

SELF-RETAINING URETERAL STENTS

Self-retaining ureteral stents can be employed to dilate the ureter by a mechanism similar to that of ureteral catheterization. The ureteral stent is passed by standard techniques.[7] We prefer to pass a floppy-tipped guidewire endoscopically into the renal pelvis. The self-retaining stent is then advanced over the guidewire, and the pigtails are allowed to curl in the renal pelvis and the bladder (Fig. 5–3). The patient can then remain ambulatory and be treated as an outpatient as the ureter is dilated with the stent in place.

The self-retaining stent technique is excellent for long, narrow areas or strictures within the ureter. It also allows resolution of massive edema

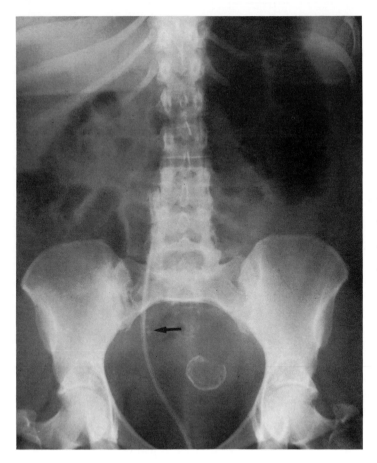

Figure 5–2. Three catheters have been placed into the right ureter to dilate the orifice and distal ureter and to drain urine proximal to the obstructing calculus (arrow). The large calcification in the left pelvis was located in a uterine myoma and was unrelated to the patient's calculus.

surrounding a ureteral calculus. There may be some additional edema within the bladder from the distal pigtail of the catheter but this is usually considerably less than that observed with the combined ureteral catheter and Foley catheter.

Acute Techniques for Dilation

The ureterovesical junction can be dilated acutely, at the time of the ureteropyeloscopic procedure. Several different techniques have been described, each providing satisfactory results and having its own advantages and disadvantages. Dilation has been performed with unguided instruments passed directly under vision into the ureteral orifice and also with instruments passed over an intra-ureteral guidewire.

ACUTE URETERAL DILATION WITH CATHETERS

The ureteral orifice can be dilated by passing successively larger catheters cystoscopically into the ureteral orifice. The orifice is first examined cysto-

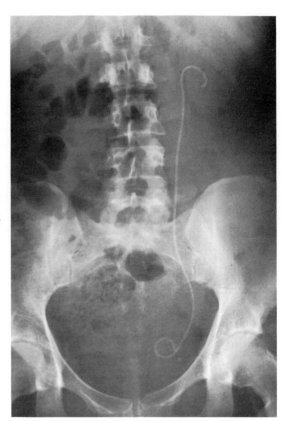

Figure 5–3. A double pigtail catheter has been placed into the ureter to dilate a narrow segment approximately 6 cm. in length and to provide drainage of urine from that kidney.

scopically, and the selected ureteral catheter is passed into the ureter for approximately 4 to 6 cm. to assure its placement through the entire intramural portion of the ureter. That catheter is then removed entirely and the next larger catheter (1 or 2 F sizes larger) is similarly passed into the orifice. This technique is limited by the size of catheter that can be passed through the cystoscope. This is usually 9 to 12 F, which may not provide adequate dilation. Any type of ureteral catheter can be employed. Olive- or round-tipped catheters are less likely to injure the ureteral mucosa than whistle-tipped catheters. Cone-tipped or Braasch bulb catheters can also be employed and are not limited by the size of the shaft within the bridge of the cystoscope. Thus, dilation to 12 or even 14 F, may be possible with cone-tipped catheters. The tips of these catheters are often relatively sharp and may perforate the ureter.

Cone-Shaped Metal Bougie Dilators

Metal cone-tipped dilators have been used with considerable success for dilating the ureterovesical junction. Cone-tipped dilators were described as early as 1924,[2] for dilation of the ureter to facilitate passage of calculi or urine. Lyon's early reports of ureteroscopy included a description of metal cone-tipped ureteral dilators.[4] Although the original instruments had interchangeable tips, the presently available dilators consist of a cone-shaped metal tip attached to a flexible carrier. Tips are available in sizes from 10 to 15 F (Fig. 5–4).

The ureter is dilated endoscopically. After the orifice has been identified cystoscopically, the smallest ureteral dilator (10 F) is passed into the orifice under direct vision and advanced along the course of the ureter until it can be felt to pass through the intramural portion into the more proximal ureter (Fig. 5–5). The larger dilators are successively passed in a similar fashion. The larger (15 F) dilator must be backloaded into the standard cystoscopic bridge. Thus, after the previous dilator has been removed from the cysto-scope, the telescope and the bridge are removed from the sheath of the cystoscope. The back, or handle portion, of the dilator is then passed in a retrograde fashion through the bridge of the cystoscope. The tip is allowed to protrude beyond the tip of the telescope itself. The entire assembled unit, bridge with telescope and dilator, is then replaced in the sheath. Under direct vision, the largest dilator can then be passed into the ureter and along the intramural portion.

Because of the increased risk of perforation due to misdirection of the conical dilators, it is essential to align the dilator and cystoscope along the projected three-dimensional course of the intramural ureter. To approximate this course, an imaginary line is extended from the center of the ureteral lumen (see Fig. 5–5). The cystoscope and dilator are then aligned along the line.

Since these dilators are not guided, they are likely to cause perforation (Fig. 5–6). Perforation usually occurs either laterally or medially within the intramural portion of the ureter. Medial perforation may cause the dilator to re-enter the bladder, whereas a lateral course can bring the dilator into the perivesical space. Although it is not systemically serious and does not result in a urinoma, if the ureter is not properly drained intraluminally, perforation may impede or prevent the ureteropyeloscopic procedure (see subsequent section).

GUIDED DILATORS

Several techniques for ureteral dilation employ an angiographic guide-wire within the ureter. There is less potential for ureteral perforation with these techniques, since the less traumatic guidewire is first placed into the ureter and then the dilating instruments are advanced into the ureter over the guidewire. At the completion of dilation, the guidewire is left within the ureter to facilitate placement of the ureteropyeloscope under vision into the orifice. These techniques may be impossible if a guidewire cannot be passed into the ureter. Although prevention of guidewire passage is unusual, it may occur with a distal calculus or with a calculus within the intramural tunnel. When possible, the guided techniques are preferred for dilation of the ureterovesical junction.

FLEXIBLE GRADUATED DILATORS

Flexible dilators, similar to those used for dilating the tract for percu-taneous nephrostomy, are available in a suitable length (70 cm.) and sizes (8

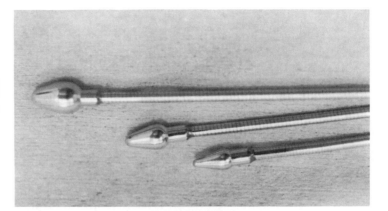

Figure 5–4. The cone-shaped metal bougie dilators are passed into the ureter without guidewire control.

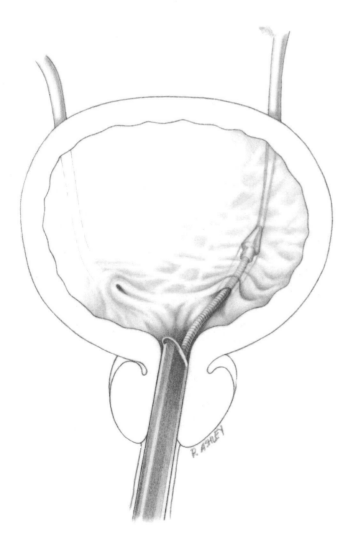

Figure 5–5. The cone-shaped dilator is advanced into the ureteral tunnel and must be carefully directed along the anticipated position of the ureteral lumen.

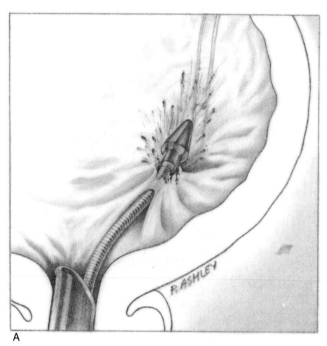

A

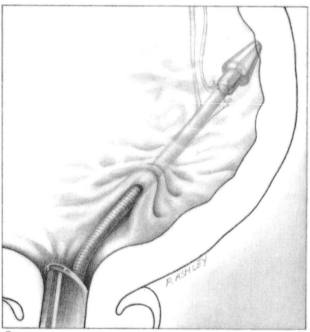

B

Figure 5–6. Misdirection of the cone-shaped dilators results in perforation of the ureteral wall. A, Medial perforation in the intravesical segment may re-enter the bladder or may course submucosally. B, Lateral perforation passes into the perivesical tissue.

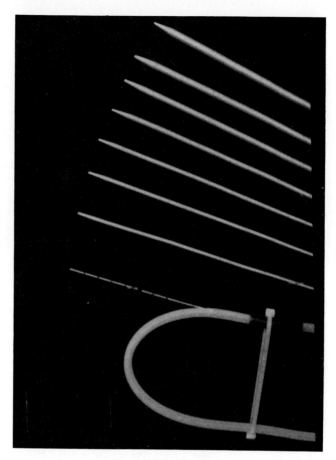

Figure 5–7. Graduated dilators have tapered tips and cylindrical bodies, and are radiopaque.

to 16 F) for ureteral dilation (Fig. 5–7). They can be used to dilate the ureterovesical junction and the distal portion of the ureter (Fig. 5–8).

After the appropriate orifice has been identified cystoscopically, a guidewire is advanced from the cystoscope into the ureteral orifice and proximally within the ureter. A 0.038-inch, straight, floppy-tipped, heavy-duty angiographic guidewire can be employed. This will usually pass easily within the ureter; the floppy tip allows the guidewire to pass the angulation of the distal ureter at the bladder. The guidewire will also usually pass a calculus without dislodging it, although fluoroscopic control helps to determine the position of the calculus during placement (see Chapter 6). The guidewire is passed to the level of the renal pelvis. If it does not pass an obstruction, such as a calculus, it can still be employed for dilation as long as several centimeters of the rigid portion of the wire are within the ureter. The flexible floppy tip cannot be employed for dilation, since it is not firm enough to guide dilators. If a stiffer wire is needed, then this standard wire can be exchanged through a catheter for a Lunderquist wire.

Some urologists have used intraluminal lubrication with 1% Xylocaine jelly to facilitate placement of the dilators. The lubricant (2 to 3 ml.) is injected into the ureteral lumen through the same catheter used for the retrograde pyelogram.

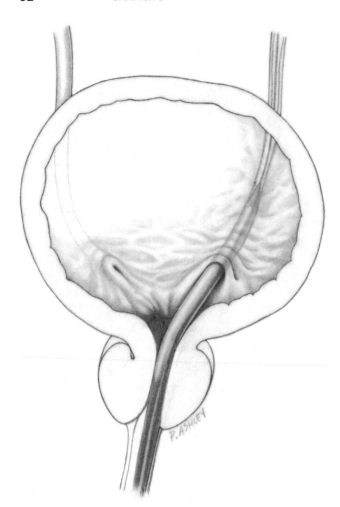

Figure 5–8. *The graduated dilator is generally used in the intramural and distal ureter but can be placed more proximally with fluoroscopic control when necessary.*

After the guidewire has been appropriately placed, the smallest dilator that can be easily accommodated within the ureter is passed over the guidewire through the cystoscope under direct vision into the ureteral orifice. It should be passed through the entire intramural ureter. If there is a narrow area within the distal ureter, it can also be passed within that portion. It is safest to use fluoroscopic guidance both for passing the guidewire and for passing dilators into the mid- or distal ureter. The dilator is then removed, and successively larger dilators are passed over the guidewire into the orifice and through the intramural portion.

The smaller dilators can be passed under direct vision, but visual placement is limited by the size of the dilators that can be accommodated within the cystoscope. Usually, this is 10 or 12 F. The larger dilators (i.e., 12 or 14 F) must be passed with fluoroscopic control alone. After the largest dilator that will pass through the cystoscope has been used, the telescope and bridge can be removed, leaving the guidewire within the sheath of the cystoscope, or the entire cystoscope can be removed, leaving the guidewire in place. The next larger dilator is then passed over the guidewire and observed on the fluoroscope to pass the level of the intramural ureter. This

technique obviously lacks the visual control afforded by the totally endoscopic techniques. By leaving the sheath of the cystoscope in position near
the orifice, the dilator can be guided through the bladder to enter the orifice.

DILATING SHEATH SYSTEM

A dilating sheath system, which consists of four coaxial Teflon catheters
ranging in size from 6 to 17 F, has been described.[5] The 6-F catheter is first
introduced cystoscopically into the ureteral orifice. It is advanced to the
desired level in the ureter and subsequently, the 10-F catheter is advanced
over the smaller catheter until its tip also lies at the point of interest. The
cystoscope can then be removed, and the larger catheters can be passed
coaxially over the first two. The inner catheters can then be removed, leaving
only the 17-F sheath in place. The ureteropyeloscope is then passed through
this sheath to the level of interest without specifically negotiating the urethra,
ureteral orifice, or distal ureter.

Newman and co-workers have noted some difficulty in displacing calculi
proximally into the intrarenal collecting system and in placing the sheath to
distal ureteral lesions.[5] Since the distal ureter is obscured by the sheath, the
dilator sheathing technique should be avoided when inspection of the entire
ureter is desired, such as in the investigation or treatment of ureteral filling
defects. Also, there may be some concern that leaving such a large instrument
within the ureter during the course of the procedure may cause some relative
ischemia of portions of the ureter. Certainly, when working within the
urethra (such as during resection of the prostate), it is advantageous to use
the smallest instrument possible to avoid stricture formation. These authors,
however, have observed no ureteral strictures in their relatively short period
of follow up. We have not had experience with this technique but rather
have preferred to limit dilation to the intramural ureter and other sites as
necessary.

DILATING BALLOON CATHETERS

Balloon catheters similar to angioplastic balloon catheters have been
adapted for ureteral dilation. These catheters are available in 4.5 to 7 F
diameters with an inflated balloon diameter of 5 and 6 mm. and lengths
from 3 to 10 cm. Other catheters are available with diameters of 7 or 8 mm.
and lengths approaching that of the entire ureter.

The dilating balloon catheter can be placed in the orifice directly or,
preferably, over a guidewire. The catheter can be positioned most accurately
with less chance of perforation by passing it over a guidewire. The standard
0.038-inch floppy-tipped guidewire is passed cystoscopically into the ureter.
The balloon catheter is then advanced over the guidewire through the
cystoscope into the orifice under endoscopic visual control. The balloon is
positioned to allow full dilation of the ureteral orifice and the intramural
ureter. Therefore, the first dilation should be performed with the balloon
protruding a few millimeters from the orifice to be certain that the orifice is
dilated by the cylindrical portion of the inflated balloon (Fig. 5–9). If a short
balloon is employed, then it should be advanced after deflating and re-

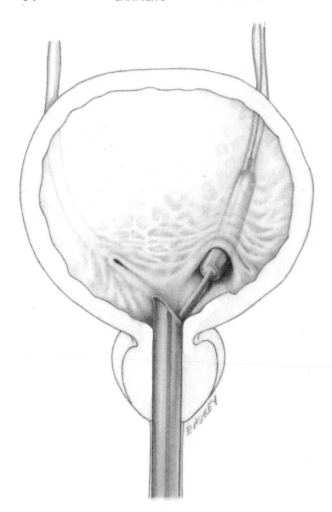

Figure 5–9. A balloon dilating catheter should be placed so that the entire intramural ureter and ureteral orifice are dilated. The proximal cylindrical portion of the balloon should appear in the ureteral orifice.

inflated to dilate the entire intramural ureter. With the longer (10 cm.) balloon, a single placement can provide adequate dilation of the entire appropriate segment of ureter.

The balloon is inflated with the appropriate volume of fluid under pressure as described for the individual balloon. We prefer to use a dilute solution of radiographic contrast medium (30%) for inflating the balloon and to follow the positioning and inflation fluoroscopically to assure full dilation without persistent waisting, indicating failure to dilate a segment (Fig. 5–10).

Some apparently normal ureters contain short segments that require high pressures for dilation. Although we have been able to dilate more than 60 per cent of ureterovesical junctions with a pressure of 4 atmospheres or less, approximately 10 per cent required up to 12 atmospheres, and a few required 16 or more atmospheres.[8] We now routinely use balloon catheters capable of expansion to pressures of 16 atmospheres.

The major advantages of balloon dilation are the ease and speed of the dilating process as well as the capability of dilating the ureter at any level. The small balloons, which can be passed through the ureteropyeloscope, can

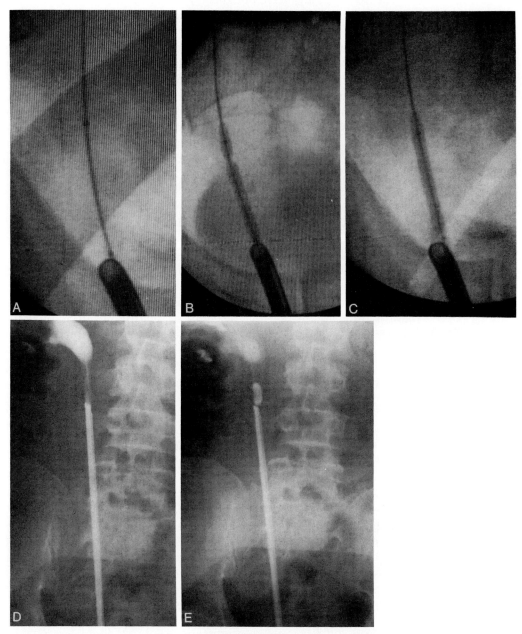

Figure 5–10. A, *Fluoroscopic views of the dilating balloon catheter with the radiopaque markers positioned at the ureterovesical junction. B, Initial inflation of the balloon leaves a narrow waist at the UVJ, indicating incomplete dilation. C, The pressure within the balloon can be increased within the limits for that particular balloon to dilate that segment as well. D, A 48-year-old patient was evaluated ureteroscopically for a filling defect in the middle infundibulum of the right kidney. An area of narrowing was encountered near the ureteropelvic junction which would not permit passage of the instrument into the renal pelvis. E, Under endoscopic vision, a 4 mm. balloon on a 4.5 balloon catheter was inserted through the ureteropyeloscope and inflated at the level of the narrowing. This dilated the narrow segment and allowed the instrument to be passed into the renal pelvis.*

be inflated under direct vision and can be used throughout the ureter (see subsequent section).

The major disadvantage of balloon dilation is the cost of the catheters, which are recommended by the manufacturer for one-time use only. In our early experience with angioplastic balloon catheters, full dilation was often not achieved and it was necessary to pass a metal dilator in addition to the balloon catheter. Much of this difficulty has been overcome by using the newer high pressure balloons and by monitoring the adequacy of dilation fluoroscopically.

Latex balloon catheters such as the Fogarty catheter should not be used for ureteral dilation since the elastic balloon expands asymmetrically and bulges out of the narrow segment. The normal ureter adjacent to a structure may suffer overexpansion and even rupture as the elastic, latex balloon migrates from the narrow segment.

FASCIAL DILATING BALLOON CATHETERS

Some urologists have reported using the fascial dilating balloon catheters for ureteral dilation.[9] These balloons achieve a diameter of 8 or 10 mm. when inflated and can accept pressures of greater than 10 atmospheres. Thus, they can provide a powerful, but possibly excessively large, dilation. There is little information on the long- or short-term effects of ureteral dilation to this caliber. Since this diameter is usually considerably more than is required for endoscopic manipulation and there may be theoretical disadvantages to such large acute dilation,[10] we prefer dilation to a smaller diameter except possibly in specific instances or until long-term results indicate specific advantages.

BALLOON DILATION THROUGH THE URETEROPYELOSCOPE

The development of balloon catheters of less than 5 F with a balloon capable of inflating to 5 mm. has made it possible to dilate the ureter under vision through the ureteropyeloscope itself. This technique offers considerable time savings, since the ureter can be visualized, dilated, and entered with a single endoscope. Earlier attempts at visual dilation through the ureteropyeloscope were successful but utilized coronary angioplasty balloon catheters. Routine application of this technique was impossible because of the prohibitive cost of the catheters. The development of reliable small-diameter balloon catheters has now made this technique a reality.

The ureteropyeloscope is passed transurethrally, and the orifice is visualized. The balloon catheter, which has been passed through the ureteropyeloscope, is then advanced into the orifice and positioned so that the cylindrical portion of the balloon extends from the orifice itself. The balloon is then inflated with dilute radiographic contrast material so that the adequacy of dilation can be followed radiographically. If a narrow waist is formed in the balloon indicating an undilated segment, then another technique for dilation may be needed to assure full dilation. After the balloon has been fully expanded, it is deflated. It may be necessary to aspirate the fluid from the balloon with a syringe because of the small lumen within the catheter.

Total collapse of the balloon can be confirmed visually and radiographically. As the balloon is withdrawn into the ureteropyeloscope, the instrument can be advanced immediately into the orifice. If more proximal portions of the ureter require dilation, then the procedure can be repeated at those levels, and the adequacy of dilation can be followed visually (see Fig. 5–10C and D).

Particular care must be taken to assure that the balloon is fully deflated before attempting to withdraw it into the sheath of the ureteropyeloscope. Since there is very fine tolerance between the lumen of the working channel in the instrument and the balloon catheter, any fluid left within the balloon may exceed this tolerance and lead to damage to the balloon itself.

Some urologists prefer to examine the bladder with a cystoscope first and place a guidewire into the ureteral orifice in the usual fashion. The guidewire can then remain during the ureteropyeloscopic procedure as a safety precaution and can be available for placement of a ureteral catheter. Examination of the bladder with a standard cystoscope also provides greater visibility with better illumination and a wider field of vision than that obtained through the ureteropyeloscope alone.

OLIVE-TIPPED METAL DILATORS

Flexible metal dilators that accept a guidewire and have an olive-shaped tip have proved exceptionally useful for ureteral dilation. The particular shape of the tip, with a smoothly rounded proximal and distal design, allows for easy passage and removal from the ureteral orifice (Fig. 5–11). Fabrication of metal assures full dilation of the lumen to the diameter of the dilator and also provides clear visualization radiographically. These dilators are reusable and can be sterilized in an autoclave.

The olive-tipped dilators can be used with or without a guidewire. Passage over a guidewire minimizes the chance for perforation. The standard 0.038-inch, straight, floppy-tipped angiographic guidewire is placed endoscopically into the ureteral orifice and advanced to the level of the renal pelvis. The smallest of the dilators, which range from 8 to 16 F, is then

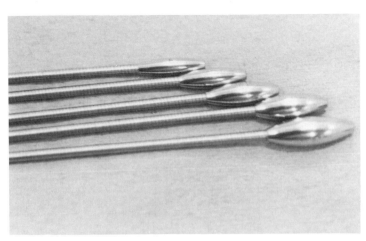

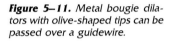
Figure 5–11. Metal bougie dilators with olive-shaped tips can be passed over a guidewire.

passed over the guidewire through the cystoscope and into the orifice under visual control. It is passed through the entire intramural portion of the ureter (Fig. 5–12). If it is necessary to dilate a proximal segment of the ureter, then the dilator can be passed under fluoroscopic control through that segment of the ureter as well (Fig. 5–13). Proximal dilation should be attempted only when the dilator is being passed with a guidewire.

The larger dilators, 14 and 16 F, must be backloaded into the cystoscope, since they will not pass through the bridge or the sheath with a telescope in place. In order to position these dilators, the telescope and bridge are removed from the sheath, but the guidewire is left in place. The larger dilator is then placed over the guidewire, and the wire and handle of the dilator are passed in a retrograde fashion through the bridge. The tip of the dilator is positioned beyond the objective tip of the telescope, and the entire unit—dilator, bridge, and telescope—is repositioned in the sheath. The larger dilator can then be advanced in position over the guidewire into the ureter with visual control. At the completion of dilation, the guidewire can be left in position and the dilator and cystoscope removed.

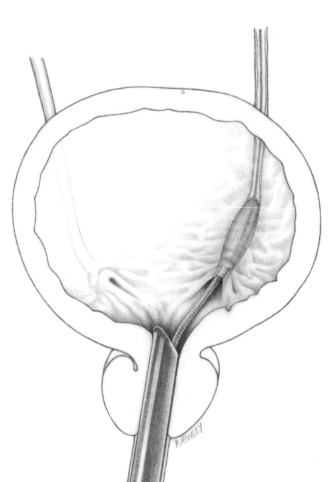

Figure 5–12. Metal bougie dilators are generally passed through the intramural ureter over the guidewire for dilation.

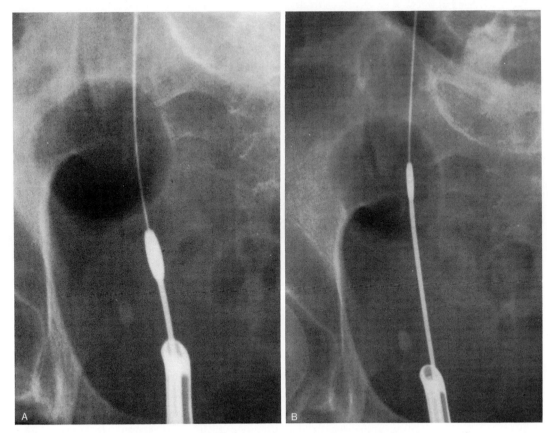

Figure 5–13. A and B, *These metal bougie dilators can be passed more proximally in the ureter if necessary, since they have excellent tactile control and are readily seen on the fluoroscope.*

SPECIAL DILATING PROBLEMS

Although most ureters can be readily dilated to accept the ureteropyeloscope, in certain situations particular difficulty may be anticipated. The ureteral orifice that is inaccessible to the cystoscopic approach obviously cannot be instrumented for dilation. This has occurred rarely in patients with severe prostatic enlargement. The orifice may also be inaccessible after re-implantation. This and other surgical procedures may also cause scarring of the ureterovesical junction, which is then difficult to dilate. The greatest success in this situation has been with high pressure balloon catheters. Dilation may also be assisted by placement of an indwelling ureteral catheter or stent.

One of the major difficulties in dilating occurs with a calculus impacted in the distal ureter at the ureterovesical junction. Often in such cases a guidewire cannot be passed. It is then necessary to dilate with the unguided metal dilators to the level of the calculus. The operating ureteropyeloscope with offset telescope is then most effectively used to approach the calculus and fragment it under direct vision. Alternatively, a balloon catheter with a very short tip, or no tip, can be used and placed to the level of the calculus for dilation. Some of the smaller diameter endoscopes can be placed into the undilated ureter and used to position a guidewire for subsequent dilation, or with the appropriate endoscope, they can be used to fragment the calculus under vision.

Complications

INADEQUATE DILATION

Failure to dilate the ureter adequately is the most frequent problem encountered. Inadequate dilation can be recognized during the attempt at passing the ureteropyeloscope. A non-dilated segment of the intramural ureter may not accept the ureteropyeloscope; this segment moves with the instrument as it is advanced toward the lumen. Repeated attempts at passage of the endoscope do not dilate the ureter, and it is essential to remove the instrument and redilate the ureter to be certain that the dilating instrument passes proximally through that segment. If the narrow segment can be seen with the ureteropyeloscope, then a balloon catheter passed through the instrument under vision is an excellent technique for dilating.

PERFORATION

Perforation of the ureteral mucosa is an uncommon complication when dilation is performed with one of the guided techniques. It is seen more frequently when one of the unguided techniques is used. In those cases, perforation is usually in the medial or lateral aspect of the intravesical ureter, just as it enters the vesical musculature. Adequate drainage must be achieved, usually with a ureteral catheter, which can be placed easily if a guidewire has been placed. Inadequate drainage may result in a urinoma and infectious sequelae (Fig. 5–14).

MIGRATION OF CALCULUS

During the dilation of a ureter that contains a stone near the uretero-vesical junction, contact between the dilating instrument or the guidewire and the calculus may force the calculus more proximally within the ureter (see Chapter 6). Every attempt should be made to avoid moving the calculus significantly more proximally within the ureter. If it is impossible to place a guidewire beyond the calculus, then it may be necessary to dilate the ureterovesical junction or at least the distal intravesical ureter with one of the unguided techniques, such as the use of the metal cone-tipped dilators. For a more proximally located calculus, care should be taken to avoid passing the dilator to the stone itself in order to prevent proximal migration.

In certain cases, particularly those in which the calculus is located directly at the ureterovesical junction, it may even prove advantageous to move the calculus proximally into the more dilated distal ureter. However, special care should be taken to keep the calculus distal to the iliac vessels. In that position within the distal ureter it may be easier to place a basket or other device on the calculus for withdrawing or fragmenting the stone.

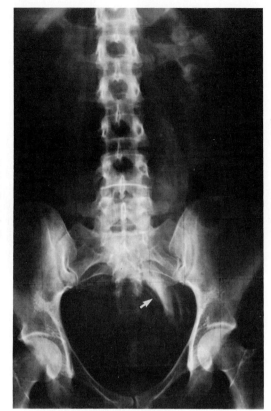

Figure 5–14. In this patient, the left distal ureter was dilated with a balloon catheter without the benefit of a guidewire. The urologist was unable to pass the instrument after the dilation and could not pass a ureteral catheter. An excretory urogram demonstrated extravasation of contrast from the level of the distal ureter tracking along the ureter superiorly as shown in this radiograph.

OBLITERATION OF UROTHELIAL LESIONS

Since the diagnosis of filling defects requires direct observation of the untraumatized lesion, it is essential to avoid damaging the filling defect itself during dilation before endoscopic inspection. Therefore, if a filling defect within the distal ureter is to be examined, one of the unguided techniques may be preferred for ureteral dilation. For a more proximal lesion, if a guidewire is used, it should be placed distal to the lesion. In either case, the dilator should not be passed to the level of the area to be inspected in order to avoid damaging the lesion—either removing it or starting bleeding that would render it unrecognizable.

STRICTURE

Ureteral stricture is a serious potential complication. Although it bears significant consequences and may require either dilation or even re-implantation of the ureter into the bladder for treatment, it is a rare complication. Although sporadic occurrences have been reported, in our series numbering over 300 patients, no ureterovesical junction strictures have yet been identified. Because of the lack of experience with this problem, causal factors have not been determined.

In general, it would seem prudent to follow guidelines for avoiding urethral strictures. Undue ureteral trauma should be avoided, but dilation should be continued to the extent necessary for easy placement of the instrument, and the smallest instrument practical should be used. It also may be desirable to limit the length of the procedure, particularly when it has been difficult to dilate the ureter.

REFLUX

Vesicoureteral reflux has been considered a potential complication. Any inflammation or scarring of the ureterovesical junction can result in reflux as is seen with urinary tract infections. In a search for this complication clinically, Lyon examined 15 patients with cystography following dilation for ureteropyeloscopy and found no instances of reflux.[4] Ford and co-workers performed intravenous urograms and micturating cystograms three months after ureteroscopy with dilation of the ureterovesical junction to 14 F. Grade I vesicoureteral reflux was detected in a single patient without evidence of other abnormalities. The same authors found little histologic or radiologic alteration of ureters of rabbits dilated to 4 F (threefold). However, dilation to 7 F produced partial ureterovesical junction obstruction with histologic evidence of disruption and fibrosis.[11]

From the available evidence, dilation of the human ureter to approximately 15 F is not detrimental to its integrity or function. Use of this procedure in several hundred patients has not been found to be detrimental.

References

1. Lewis B: Discussion. Trans Am Assoc GU Surg 1:124, 1906.
2. Dourmashkin RL: Cystoscopic treatment of stones in the ureter with special reference to large calculi: based on the study of 1550 cases. J Urol 54:245, 1945.
3. Dourmashkin RL: Dilatation of the ureter with rubber bags in the treatment of ureteral calculi. Presentation of a modified operating cystoscope. A preliminary report. J Urol 15:449, 1926.
4. Lyon ES, Kyker JS, and Schoenberg HW: Transurethral ureteroscopy in women: a ready addition to urologic armamentarium. J Urol 119:35, 1978.
5. Newman RC, Hunter PT, Hawkins IF, and Finlayson B: A general ureteral dilator-sheathing system. Urology 25:287, 1985.
6. Perez-Castro Ellendt E and Martinez-Pineiro JA: Transurethral ureteroscopy—a current urological procedure. Arch Esp Urol 33:445, 1980.
7. Huffman JL, Bagley DH, and Lyon ES: Ureteral catheterization, retrograde ureteropyelography and self-retaining ureteral stents. In Bagley DH, Huffman JL, and Lyon ES (eds.): Urologic Endoscopy: A Manual and Atlas. Boston, Little, Brown and Company, 1985, pp. 163–176.
8. Bagley DH and Huffman JL: Balloon dilation of the ureterovesical junction: pressure requirements. (unpublished data)
9. Daughtry JD, Bean WJ, Rodan BA, and Mullin DM: Balloon dilation of the urether: a means to facilitate passage of ureteral and renal calculi. J Urol 136:1063, 1986.
10. Greene LF: The renal and ureteral changes induced by dilating the ureter. An experimental study. J Urol 52:505, 1944.
11. Ford TF, Constance Parkinson M, and Wickham JEA: Clinical and experimental evaluation of ureteric dilatation. Br J Urol 56:460, 1984.

CHAPTER 6

Technique of Transurethral Passage of the Rigid Ureteropyeloscope

JEFFRY L. HUFFMAN
DEMETRIUS H. BAGLEY

The technique for insertion of the ureteropyeloscope is not unlike other endoscopic procedures, which are very familiar to urologists. The rigid instruments and sheaths are identical to pediatric endoscopes except for the added length. The basic process of direct vision insertion into the ureter is similar to insertion of the cystoscope through the urethra.

The previous chapters have outlined two essential components of the technique: preoperative preparation and dilation of the intramural ureter. This chapter discusses the actual process of insertion of the ureteroscope, including conventional passage, which is possible in the majority of procedures, and the more difficult procedures in which the urologist must improvise to secure passage. Although there are many variations of this technique currently in use, we will describe our experience, which has led to successful results and few complications in a high percentage of patients.[1, 2, 3, 4]

Positioning the Patient for Transurethral Ureteroscopy

A standard dorsal lithotomy position is used to begin a ureteroscopic procedure. Occasionally, variations in position are needed for procedures involving ureteral or renal pelvic calculi to ensure that gravitational forces help keep the stone in the most dependent position of the collecting system and help prevent proximal stone migration.

It is desirable to hyperabduct the patient's contralateral hip prior to beginning the procedure. This enables the instrument to attain an angle closest to that of the intramural ureter as it is inserted. The angle is best approximated by extending a line that bisects the center of the intramural ureteral lumen (Fig. 6–1).

Passing the instrument above the level of the pelvic brim can usually be achieved with the patient horizontal. However, as the renal pelvis is approached, a Trendelenburg position allows the entire kidney to take a more superior position, thus straightening the proximal ureter and the ureteropelvic junction. Once the ureteropyeloscope is within the renal pelvis, different patient positions are used to help view the various infundibula. In these instances, a table with controls to tilt the patient in three planes is desirable.

Other variations in position are often used, depending on problems that are encountered intra-operatively. These are discussed in detail in a later section.

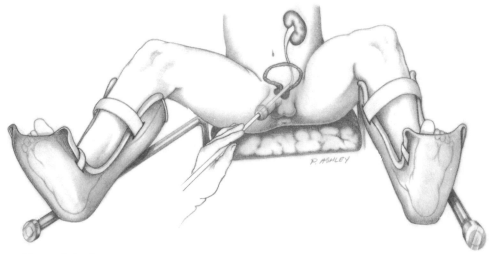

Figure 6–1. *The patient's contralateral hip is abducted to enable an angle of insertion of the ureteropyeloscope that closely approximates the three-dimensional plane of the intramural ureter.*

Fluid for Irrigation During Ureteroscopy

Special irrigating fluids are not required for a ureteroscopic procedure and those used for transurethral surgery within the bladder are employed. For diagnostic ureteroscopy and stone removal normal saline irrigant is utilized. This approximates a physiologic solution, which is important in the event irrigant is absorbed into the circulation following inadvertent perforation of the collecting system or pyelorenal backflow.

Glycine is used as irrigation only for ureteroscopic electrosurgery. Initially, saline is used, and immediately prior to the electrosurgical part of the procedure, the irrigation fluid is switched to glycine. Although water can also be employed, glycine is preferred because it has osmolality similar to that of the circulation and thus is non-hemolytic.

The pressure of the irrigating fluid is significant. We recognized the significance after many patients complained of flank pain following ureteroscopic procedures. This was thought to be due to overdistension of the intrarenal collecting system. Since we now limit the height of the irrigant to 30 cm., the post-operative finding of flank pain has diminished.

Insertion of the Ureteropyeloscope

The technique for passage of the rigid ureteropyeloscope is very similar to that used for urethroscopy, and similar precautions are necessary (Table 6–1). In general these include: (1) direct vision during insertion into the ureter, keeping the lumen centered in the viewing field, (2) proximal advancement only when the lumen is clearly visualized, and (3) proximal

Table 6–1

GUIDELINES FOR SUCCESSFUL TRANSURETHRAL
URETEROPYELOSCOPY

1. Direct visual passage of the ureteropyeloscope into the bladder and ureter, keeping the lumen within the viewing field.
2. Proximal advancement within the ureter only when the lumen is well visualized.
3. Proximal advancement only if the tip of the instrument slides freely along the ureteral wall and does not bind.

advancement only when the instrument beak slides freely along the ureteral wall and does not bind.

The instrument, with a forward viewing (0 or 5 degree) lens, is inserted under direct vision through the urethra and into the bladder. Blind insertion with an obturator is not possible because of the longer length and small diameter of the instrument. The telescope is also smaller in diameter than a standard cystoscope (2.3 to 2.7 mm.), approximately the same as a pediatric endoscope. Thus, the field of vision is smaller, often making it difficult to identify landmarks that have been defined cystoscopically. It is often helpful to leave a guidewire or catheter in the orifice following dilation to enable quick and easy identification of the orifice.

Once the ureteral orifice is identified, the instrument is aligned along the projected course of the intramural ureter (see Fig. 6–1). The orifice is approached, with the tip of the instrument directed toward the center of the lumen. At a point just outside the orifice, the instrument can be rotated 180 degrees, advanced within the os, and then returned to its upright position within the intramural ureter (Fig. 6–2). This maneuver allows the beveled tip of the instrument to slip smoothly underneath the superior margin of the orifice, and although it is not mandatory, it often facilitates insertion.

Alternatively, the tip of the instrument can be advanced directly toward the orifice and placed into the lumen to lift the overhanging mucosa. If a guidewire is in place, it can be used to lift the anterior ureteral wall with the tip of the endoscope.

Once within the intramural ureter, the instrument is advanced proximally, keeping the lumen centered in the viewing field. In order to anticipate the normal curvature of the ureter and facilitate instrument passage, it is helpful to envision the three-dimensional anatomy of the upper urinary tract (Figs. 3–1 and 3–2). As one proceeds superiorly away from the bladder, the ureter is seen to course laterally and slightly posteriorly for several centimeters before bending medially and anteriorly toward the pelvic brim. Its superior course continues across the iliac vessels, becomes essentially horizontal over the psoas muscle, and then courses posteriorly and laterally toward the renal pelvis, which actually lies at a 70-degree angle with the coronal axis of the body.[5]

Several landmarks are identifiable during passage of the instrument into the renal pelvis.[4] The intramural ureter is the narrowest part of the upper urinary tract, and its proximal margin is identified as a junction with the larger and easily distensible supravesical ureter. The transmitted pulsations of the hypogastric and common iliac arteries are seen posteromedially in the lower ureter, signifying their close proximity at this level. Two landmarks help designate the region of the proximal ureter or ureteropelvic junction:

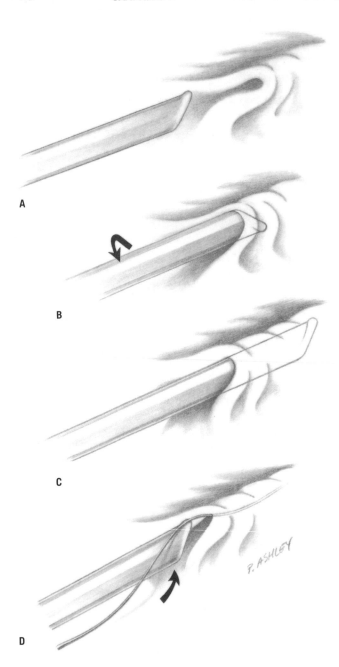

A

B

C

D

Figure 6–2. The instrument is directed toward the ureteral orifice (A). At a point just outside of the os, the instrument is rotated 180 degrees, enabling the beak of the beveled instrument to slide smoothly under the upper lip of the orifice (B). Once inside the intramural ureter, the instrument is returned to its upright position (C). If a guidewire is in place, the tip of the endoscope may be placed to lift the overhanging ureteral orifice (D).

the respiratory movement and the unique configuration of the ureter. The middle ureter is relatively fixed compared to the mobile proximal ureter, renal pelvis, and kidney. Thus, with each respiratory inspiration and downward movement of the diaphragm, the renal pelvis and proximal ureter are seen to move down also. At this junction between the fixed and mobile portions of the ureter, there is a unique anatomic configuration within the ureteral lumen. It appears as a mucosal band across the posterolateral margin of the lumen that accentuates with each bend in the ureter. As the instrument passes through this region, the more voluminous renal pelvis is visualized in the distance.

Problems Occasionally Encountered During Ureteropyeloscope Passage

The majority of patients (>90%) have upper tract collecting systems that are easily accessible with the ureteroscope[1]; however, there are occasional problems encountered in passing the instrument (Table 6–2). These problems include: (1) poor visualization, (2) upper tract narrowings, and (3) ureteral tortuosity. Although these problems do necessitate additional time for the procedure, they can usually be conquered using a variety of techniques familiar to most urologic endoscopists. The urologist must realize, however, that an occasional patient will have an anatomic configuration that will not allow passage of a rigid ureteroscope. In these instances, the procedure must be aborted and an alternative method, such as flexible ureteropyeloscopy, must be used.

POOR VISUALIZATION

The greatest advantage of the ureteroscopic technique is direct visual access to the ureter and pelvis. When visualization is impaired secondary to bleeding, edema, or inflammatory debris, the endoscopic advantage is lost and the procedure becomes more likely to result in complications.

The initial step in overcoming the problem of poor visualization from debris or blood is to use copious amounts of irrigation through the instrument sheath without the telescope. This requires considerable time since the upper tract volume is only 5 to 10 ml.; this amount is allowed to run through the sheath and then drain by gravity until the return irrigant becomes clear.

Table 6–2
PROBLEMS OCCASIONALLY ENCOUNTERED DURING
PASSAGE OF THE URETEROPYELOSCOPE

Problem	Solution
1. Poor visualization (blood, debris)	1. Persistent irrigation and drainage through sheath alone 2. Hand irrigation through 4-F catheter 3. High-pressure irrigation through syringe 4. Use of continuous flow sheath
2. Ureteral narrowing or stricture	1. Balloon dilation through sheath 2. Dilation with guided, olive-tipped bougies cystoscopically 3. Dilation with 70-cm. graduated dilators 4. Insertion of an indwelling ureteral stent
3. Ureteral tortuosity	1. Place patient in steep Trendelenburg position 2. Pass catheter or guidewire to straighten ureter

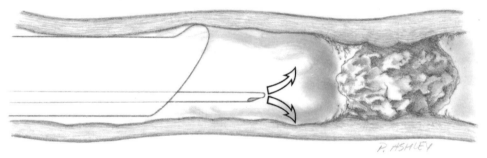

Figure 6–3. *Blood or debris within the ureter hampers visualization and should be cleared before the instrument is advanced. A 4 F catheter is passed and positioned at the tip of the instrument. Gentle hand irrigation through this catheter will provide clear vision immediately ahead of the instrument and allow safe advancement.*

Another solution to the problem of poor visualization involves passing a 4-F whistle-tipped or open-ended catheter so that its tip is located at the beak of the instrument. An assistant mechanically irrigates through the catheter using a 5-ml. syringe. This clears the view at the tip of the instrument, enabling visualization of the lumen and safe proximal advancement of the instrument (Fig. 6–3). Use of the constant flow sheath provides the same benefit.

High pressure irrigation is also helpful. A Luer-Lok tip syringe (20 to 50 ml.) is attached directly to the irrigation port of the ureteroscope. Pulses of irrigation from the syringe often provide the necessary clear field of view. Certain precautions must be taken when using this method. Clearly, high pressure may cause proximal stone migration or overdistension of the upper tract. The stone's position should be monitored fluoroscopically, and the upper tract should be emptied intermittently.

UPPER TRACT NARROWING

Occasionally as the instrument is inserted, the lumen is clearly visible; however, its size is not sufficient to allow passage of the instrument. These regions of narrowing or non-distensible bands within the ureter are not usually associated with proximal distension of the urinary tract and thus cannot be termed pathologic strictures. However, they do impede instrument passage and must be dealt with in a manner so as not to cause complications.

These regions are easily recognized. Instead of smoothly sliding along the ureteral wall, the tip of the instrument will cause telescoping of the ureter (Fig. 6–4). Persisting with forceful instrument advancement inevitably leads to perforation or avulsion of the ureter.

The methods used to overcome these obstructions include: dilation with balloon catheters, dilation with guided, olive-shaped metal bougies, catheter dilation with 70-cm. graduated dilators, and placement of an indwelling ureteral stent. These techniques are described in detail in Chapter 5.

URETERAL TORTUOSITY

Tortuosities within the ureter without narrow regions are commonly encountered. These usually can be negotiated with the instrument; however,

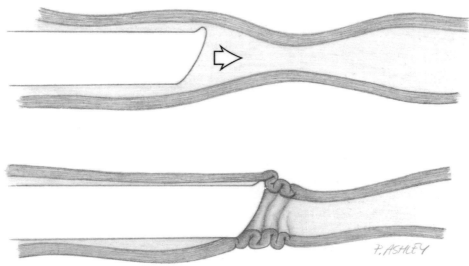

Figure 6–4. Narrowed regions within the ureter may prohibit instrument passage and must be dilated. These regions are recognized when the ureteral wall binds the tip of the ureteropyeloscope, causing telescoping of the ureter as the instrument is advanced.

there are two other methods to aid the endoscopist in these instances. The initial step is to position the patient in a steep Trendelenburg position. This allows the normally mobile kidney to assume a more superior position near the diaphragm, thus straightening the proximal ureter. This maneuver may have no effect on a previously operated kidney. If significant tortuosity remains, the second step is to pass a 4-F whistle-tipped ureteral catheter through the instrument to a position proximal to the tortuous ureteral bend. This helps straighten the ureter and allows visualization of the proximal lumen, thus enabling safe proximal passage of the instrument along the catheter. A guidewire can be used in a similar fashion.

Approximately 10 per cent of ureteroscopic procedures cannot be performed because of marked tortuosity of the urinary tract or extended regions of narrowed ureter. Any previous retroperitoneal surgery may "fix" the ureter or renal pelvis and not permit these structures to be straightened sufficiently to allow instrument passage (see Fig. 4–1). Occasionally normal anatomic variants (Fig. 6–5) prevent successful ureteroscopy. Although a flexible ureteroscope will overcome these difficulties, it is imperative for the urologist to know the limitations of the rigid instrument, otherwise complications will ensue.

The Safety Guidewire

If a guidewire has been used for dilating, it can be left in place within the ureter as a safety guidewire throughout most ureteroscopic procedures. After completion of dilation, it is left indwelling within the urethra, bladder and ureter, and the external portion is coiled and clipped to the drapes. The ureteroscope can then be placed transurethrally alongside the guidewire. Usually the ureteroscope can pass beside the guidewire in the ureter as well.

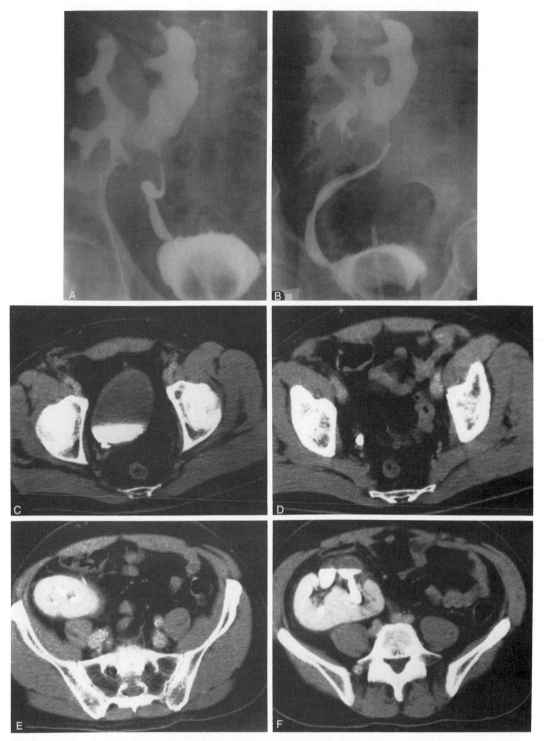

Figure 6–5. *A male patient with a crossed, fused ectopic kidney had a filling defect at the ureteropelvic junction and positive urinary cytology. A, Although the anteroposterior projection of the retrograde pyelogram shows a fairly straight ureter, the oblique projection and CT scans demonstrate the marked distance between the ureteral orifice posteriorly and the renal pelvis anteriorly (B to F). The rigid ureteropyeloscope could not be passed into the renal pelvis and the procedure was aborted.*

In particularly narrow portions, it may occlude the lumen sufficiently to make it difficult to pass the ureteroscope. These segments can then be dilated separately, or it may be preferable to withdraw the guidewire into the distal ureter beyond the narrow segment. If it has been difficult to pass the guidewire beyond a tortuous segment of the ureter or a calculus, then it may be preferable to dilate that localized ureteral segment. A guidewire may also provide a relative hindrance when attempting to engage a calculus in a basket. Care should be taken not to entrap the end of the guidewire within the basket.

Overall, the presence of a safety guidewire provides a major advantage in attaining ready access for catheter drainage of the proximal ureter and intrarenal collecting system. Even if visibility is totally lost within the lower ureter and the lumen cannot be detected to allow passage of the ureteroscope, a safety guidewire passing to the renal pelvis provides a means for establishing urinary drainage.

References

1. Huffman JL, Bagley DH, and Lyon ES: Extending cystoscopic techniques into the ureter and renal pelvis—Experience with ureteroscopy and pyeloscopy. JAMA 250:2004, 1983.
2. Lyon ES, Huffman JL, and Bagley DH: Ureteroscopy and ureteropyeloscopy. Urology 23:29, 1984.
3. Huffman JL, Bagley DH, and Lyon ES: Transurethral ureteropyeloscopy. In Bagley DH, Huffman JL, and Lyon ES (eds.): *Urologic Endoscopy—A Manual and Atlas*. Boston, Little, Brown and Company, 1985, pp. 185–206.
4. Huffman JL, Bagley DH, and Lyon ES: Technique of transureteral ureteropyeloscopy. In Clayman RV and Castameda WR (eds.): *Techniques of Endourology*. St. Louis, Washington University Press, 1984, pp. 267–294.
5. Kaye K and Goldberg ME: Applied anatomy of the kidney and ureter. Urol Clin North Am 9:3, 1982.

CHAPTER 7

Ureteropyeloscopic Removal of Upper Urinary Tract Calculi

JEFFRY L. HUFFMAN
DEMETRIUS H. BAGLEY

Probably the greatest single achievement of the ureteroscopic method has been the endoscopic removal of ureteral and renal calculi. Once thought to be absolutely "off limits" to an endoscopic approach, the entire ureter and renal pelvis have become accessible for removal of persistent calculi. As discussed in Chapter 1, initially only small distal ureteral stones were amenable to ureteroscopic removal.[1,2,3] However, the availability of the ureteropyeloscope combined with the feasibility of ultrasonic stone fragmentation eventually allowed oversized calculi, located anywhere within the ureter or renal pelvis, to be considered for endoscopic retrieval.[4]

Successful ureteropyeloscopic stone extraction depends upon proper patient selection, procedural planning, and endoscopic skill. This chapter discusses the entire stone retrieval process from the initial review of radiographic studies to the placement of ureteral catheters after the procedure, and also reviews the results of the initial experiences with these techniques.

Pre-Operative Evaluation of Radiographs

The most important study prior to ureteropyeloscopic stone manipulation is the excretory urogram. This study supplies information regarding stone location, stone size, and the degree of obstruction present. The presence of a ureteral stricture distal to the calculus or extreme tortuosity of the ureter is also determined prior to the procedure and allows better planning before ureteroscopy.

A plain radiographic film of the abdomen is taken on the operating room table prior to induction of anesthesia. It is essential for the ureteroscopist to know exactly where the calculus is located within the urinary tract at the time of the procedure. Calculi change positions rapidly, especially those that are acute and not impacted and those in a dilated ureter. A stone shown to be lodged in the mid-ureter by an excretory urogram done 24 hours earlier may have migrated proximally or distally and possibly even passed into the bladder by the time the endoscopic procedure has started.

It is valuable to have the results of a cone-tipped retrograde ureteropyelogram before approaching a calculus ureteroscopically. Often the segment of ureter distal to a calculus will not be well demonstrated on the excretory urogram. The retrograde study allows an appraisal of ureteral tortuosity and caliber prior to passing the ureteroscope, and it may identify regions within the ureter that may be difficult to negotiate. Short, non-distensible segments have frequently been identified. These must be dilated before the ureteropyeloscope is passed through the segment.

A retrograde ureteropyelogram, however, does increase the risk of displacing the calculus with the injection of contrast material. For this reason, if a retrograde ureteropyelogram is done immediately prior to the endoscopic procedure, only a small amount (3 to 5 ml.) of contrast material is instilled at very low pressure. Fluoroscopy is invaluable in these instances, since it enables continuous monitoring of the stone's position during the inflow of contrast.

Patient Positioning

The patient must be positioned so that the calculus takes a dependent position relative to the renal pelvis. Many early failures in our experience were caused by proximal stone migration. Other ureteroscopists similarly report stone migration as the prime cause of failures. Stones originally located within the ureter or pelvis are pushed with a stone basket or washed by irrigant into inaccessible locations in the kidney.

When the patient is in a supine position, any stone located in the ureter proximal to the psoas muscle is actually on a downhill slope toward the kidney (see Chapter 3). Patients with stones at this level in the ureter must be placed in a steep, reverse Trendelenburg position. Gravitational forces along with peristaltic boluses of urine will help to counteract the forces of stone basket manipulation and irrigation fluid from below.

Patients with renal pelvic calculi also need special positioning. These patients should be placed in a lateral or flank position, once again assuring dependency of the stone within the renal pelvis. The renal pelvis is located lateral and posterior to the course of the ureter (see Chapter 3). Placing the patient in a lateral position changes the position of the renal pelvis and makes it anterior relative to the ureter.

Selection of Stone Baskets and Forceps

The accessory instrument channels in most of the standard ureteropyeloscopes are 5 F. However, any bending of the instrument sheath, which often occurs during passage, has the effect of reducing the size of this working channel. Five-French accessories then become extremely snug within the instrument, making their insertion and manipulation very difficult and frustrating. Therefore, we have preferred using 4-F accessories, particularly those in Teflon sheaths to help facilitate manipulation (Fig. 7–1).

There may be two instrument channels in the working or operating ureteropyeloscope with an offset telescope. The smaller channel, which is used for stone baskets and grasping instruments when the ultrasound probe is used, is usually 4 F or smaller. Therefore, only those instruments smaller than 4 F can be used. There is a wide assortment of helical stone baskets, single and double snare designs, and three-pronged graspers available to pass through these channels.

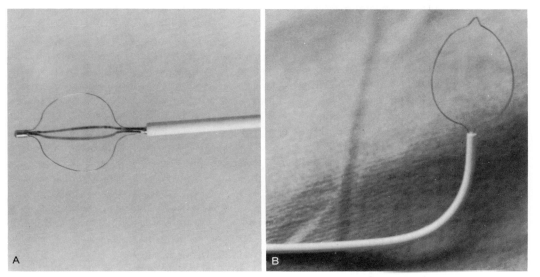

Figure 7–1. A variety of stone baskets and accessories are available for ureteroscopic stone extraction in addition to the standard Dormia or helical basket. Shown above are the 3.5 F Segura (double snare) basket (A) and the deflected 4.5 F snare (B).

Deflecting working instruments, which can be manipulated to pass laterally in the renal pelvis or even in the ureter, are also available. Single and double snares as well as three-pronged graspers are available with this design. Because of the control wire used, these instruments are necessarily larger, and at a minimum are 5 F.

The requirements of ureteroscopic stone baskets are listed in Table 7–1. Certainly, the basket must be dependable and easy to use. Non-disposable baskets often become bent, or their working mechanism becomes frozen due to excessive use and resterilization. For these reasons, the disposable baskets are preferable. Many basket designs are difficult to manipulate with only one hand. Since ureteroscopic stone manipulation is best performed by the person looking through the instrument, one-hand operation is mandatory.

A variety of basket sizes is also needed. Depending upon the size of the stone, anywhere from an 8-mm. to a 20-mm. basket diameter may be necessary. An assortment of 3-, 4-, and 6-wire baskets is also advisable.

Ureteral Dilation

Ureteral dilation is performed in a standard fashion as described in Chapter 4. However, special precautions must be taken to help prevent

Table 7–1
STONE BASKET REQUIREMENTS

Catheter size 4 F or less.
Teflon-coated catheter at least 60 cm. long.
Dependable one-hand operation.
Multiple basket sizes available.
Baskets with various numbers of wires available.

stone migration when using a guidewire method to gain adequate dilation or when approaching stones located at the ureterovesical junction or within the intramural ureter.

When using the guidewire method of dilating, there is a rule of thumb to follow for passing the guidewire. If the stone is lodged below the pelvic brim, attempt to pass the guidewire proximal to the calculus cystoscopically, but if the stone is located above the pelvic brim, pass the guidewire to a point distal to the stone. Obviously, fluoroscopic control is very useful to help guide these manipulations. Some urologists using fluoroscopy routinely pass a guidewire in all patients. It is left in place below the calculus only if it appears to move the stone or if it will not pass.

The guidewire may dislodge a stone positioned in the ureter and cause migration into the renal calyces. This is far less common with stones lodged lower than the pelvic brim, since this portion of the ureter is very dependent relative to the remainder of the collecting system. Therefore, it is advisable to pass a guidewire above stones located in these regions. This also assures that dilation will be done over the sturdy portion of the guidewire and not the less stable floppy tip.

Stones that are impacted at the ureterovesical junction or within the intramural ureter pose a difficult problem for ureteral dilation. If it is possible to pass a guidewire, dilation up to the stone generally proceeds satisfactorily. However, often with these impacted stones, it is impossible to manipulate a guidewire above the stone cystoscopically. In these instances, using the unguided conical dilators is an excellent alternative. An unguided balloon dilating catheter can also be used. The small catheters that pass through the ureteroscope offer adequate dilation, and their use allows the ureteropyeloscope to be inserted immediately after deflation of the balloon. Dilation is performed up to the stone only. Although this often leaves a segment of ureter inadequately dilated immediately distal to the stone, the dilation is usually sufficient to enable insertion of the ureteroscope. The calculus can then be visualized, and occasionally removed, without further manipulations. If a long segment of non-dilated ureter remains between the instrument tip and the stone, it is usually possible to pass a guidewire alongside the stone under vision, remove the ureteroscope, and then redilate by replacing the cystoscope and dilators, or by passing the dilators with fluoroscopic monitoring alone.

Insertion of the Ureteropyeloscope and Retrieval of Calculi

Following adequate dilation of the orifice and intramural ureter, the ureteropyeloscope is inserted. In cases in which a guidewire has been passed above the stone, it is preferable to leave the guidewire in place and pass the ureteroscope alongside the guidewire. This helps to secure the position of the calculus and facilitates insertion of the endoscope since the guidewire can be followed to locate the orifice immediately.

A stone basket can be loaded into the working channel and positioned at the end of the instrument prior to inserting the ureteropyeloscope. This allows quick and smooth advancement of the basket beyond the stone, once identified, and limits the unnecessary movement and time taken to load the basket, position it, and then re-identify the stone. Other catheters may be needed to irrigate or facilitate instrument passage, and in these instances the basket is inserted after the stone has been visualized.

As the instrument is advanced within the ureter, very little (if any) irrigation fluid should be used. Although there must be enough fluid to ensure adequate visualization of the lumen and provide adequate luminal dilation, excessive amounts of irrigant and certainly excessive pressure will only increase the chance of proximal stone migration. Even with the irrigation off, as the instrument is advanced it does push a column of fluid ahead of it. Therefore, in the ideal case, the irrigation should be off and the outflow channel should be partially open.

Often, however, there is some bleeding within the ureteral lumen from dilation, and irrigation is necessary to clear the field of view. In these patients, great care must be taken to avoid proximal displacement of the calculus. The patient should be in the reverse Trendelenburg position; the position of the calculus can be monitored intermittently fluoroscopically as the instrument is passed. Low pressure continuous flow irrigation can be obtained by inserting a ureteral catheter in the working channel of the instrument through which irrigant is passed with manual pressure on the syringe. The outflow valve of the ureteroscope is left open to provide for egress of the irrigant. Alternatively, a constant flow ureteroscope sheath can be utilized, although it is slightly larger in circumference.

Once a stone is identified, the basket should be advanced promptly beyond the stone and opened (Fig. 7–2). *This is the most critical maneuver during the procedure and must be performed smoothly and quickly.* Unnecessary instrument manipulation at this point may cause the stone to be dislodged or may cause bleeding that can obscure vision and make subsequent stone removal more difficult and possibly even dangerous.

Once the basket has been opened proximal to the stone, the stone is trapped. More irrigant can then be applied, and the full extent of the calculus appreciated. Often small blood clots are adherent to the calculus, obscuring its full extent. These can be freed by gentle to and fro washing with irrigant.

The fully opened basket is then gently withdrawn under vision alongside the calculus. The wires of the basket are then manipulated to encompass the stone. This may require several passes of the basket at several different positions in order to entrap the stone successfully. It may be helpful to open and close the basket at the level of the calculus to present the widest opening of the wires of the basket to the calculus. It is preferable for the ureteroscopist to do all the basket manipulating and not attempt to give periodic instructions to an assistant manipulating the basket. Once the wires can be visualized on opposite sides of the stone, the basket is slowly closed. As it closes, the wires are carefully observed to ensure that no mucosa becomes caught between the wires of the basket and the stone. Once the stone is secure, gentle twisting of the entire basket and stone again assures freedom within the ureter.

The stone within the basket and the instrument are then slowly removed as a unit. The basket and calculus are positioned so that the entire circumference can be seen within the ureter. The movement of the engaged calculus relative to the ureteral wall can be observed. Most stones 5 mm. or less in diameter can be removed in this fashion without further manipulation.

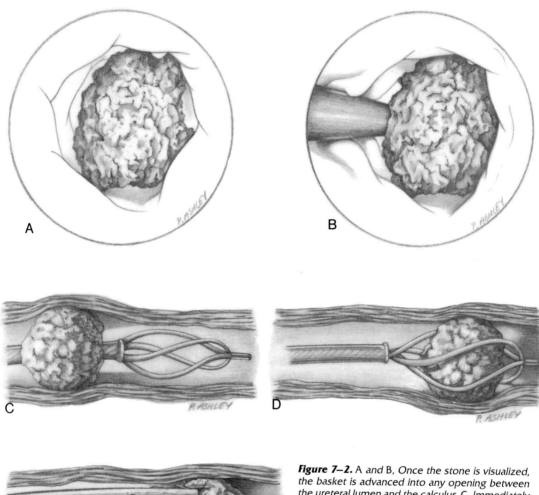

Figure 7–2. A and B, Once the stone is visualized, the basket is advanced into any opening between the ureteral lumen and the calculus. C, Immediately proximal to the stone or directly adjacent to it, the wires are opened fully and then carefully withdrawn, causing the stone to become entrapped by the basket (D). The ultrasound probe is applied to the calculus as necessary to fragment it and reduce the size for removal (E).

However, if, as the stone is removed, binding occurs between the stone and the ureteral wall, no further traction is applied (Figs. 7–3 and 7–4). One of the methods of stone fragmentation, such as ultrasonic lithotripsy, is then employed. Further traction on the basket in these instances will result in ureteral injury.[1, 4]

Removal of Large Ureteral Calculi

ULTRASONIC LITHOTRIPSY

Stones that are too large to be pulled from the ureter intact must be fragmented. Ultrasonic lithotripsy techniques, successfully used in the bladder and with percutaneous approaches, can also be directly applied ureteroscopically.[4] High frequency vibrations of a metal transducer provide the energy for stone fragmentation. The energy either fragments a stone completely or carves a path through the calculus, removing the smallest fragments by suction through its hollow central core. The transducer depends upon direct contact between its tip and the stone in order to cause fragmentation. For efficient disintegration, the stone must be secured within a basket and held in a fixed position to provide countertraction for the pressure applied to the transducer.

The ultrasonic transducer gives off heat when operating. The probe must therefore be cooled throughout the disintegration process to protect against thermal injury to the ureteral mucosa.[5] Irrigation through the ureteroscope sheath provides an excellent means of cooling and dissipation of heat. The irrigant flows in the sheath toward the tip of the probe and then flows out the ultrasonic probe suction port. It is also preferable when performing the ultrasonic fragmentation of a stone in the lower ureter to push the stone, basket, and instrument into the more proximal ureter, which is usually dilated and thus more capacious, allowing more irrigation and heat dissipation.

TECHNIQUE OF ULTRASONIC LITHOTRIPSY USING STANDARD URETEROPYELOSCOPE SHEATHS

The standard operating ureteroscopic sheaths can be effectively employed for ultrasonic lithotripsy. The disadvantage in using these sheaths rests in the need to remove the direct viewing telescope to allow room for passage of the ultrasonic transducer. The procedure is then followed audibly, fluoroscopically, and with tactile control.

The step-by-step method is outlined in Table 7–2 and depicted radiographically in Figure 7–3. Basically, while watching endoscopically, the ureteroscopist pulls the stone against the tip of the instrument. The calculus should nearly fill the entire visual field and occlude the end of of the sheath. Thus, when the direct viewing telescope is removed and replaced with the ultrasound probe, it will touch the calculus at the end of the sheath. The basket is held in this position, fixing the stone's position for ultrasonic fragmentation. At this point, the telescope is removed. The ultrasonic probe

Text continued on page 98

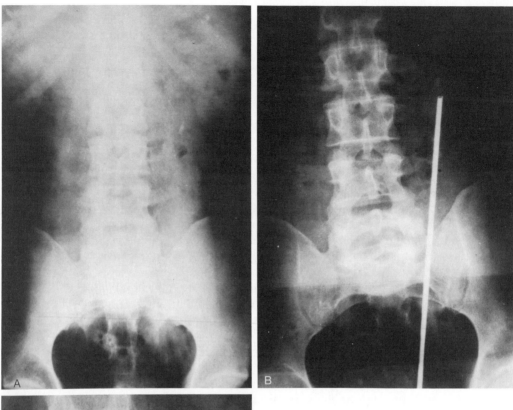

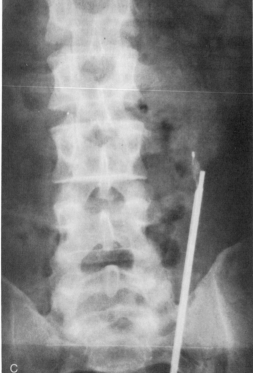

Figure 7–3. *Technique of ureteropyeloscopic ultra-sonic lithotripsy. A, A plain film of the abdomen showing a 10 × 6 mm. calculus in the proximal left ureter. B, The ureteropyeloscope is inserted, and the calculus is engaged in a stone basket under direct vision. C, If the standard ureteroscopic sheath is employed, the telescope is removed and the ultra-sonic transducer inserted to fragment the calculus. When using the offset viewing ureteroscope, the 1.5 mm. probe is inserted and fragmentation is done under vision.*

Illustration continued on opposite page

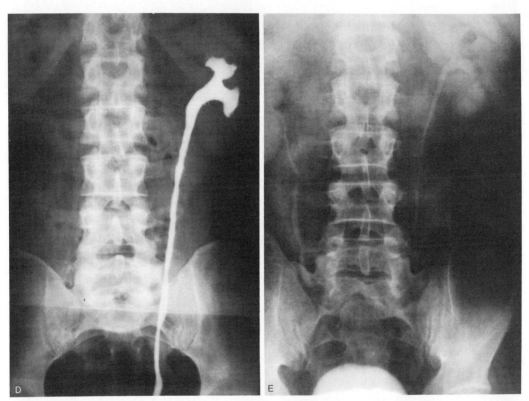

Figure 7–3 Continued D, *Following partial fragmentation in this patient, the stone could be removed. A retrograde study was performed to ensure that the ureter was intact and that no obstruction existed. E, Three months following the procedure, an excretory urogram was done to insure normal upper tract anatomy and function.*

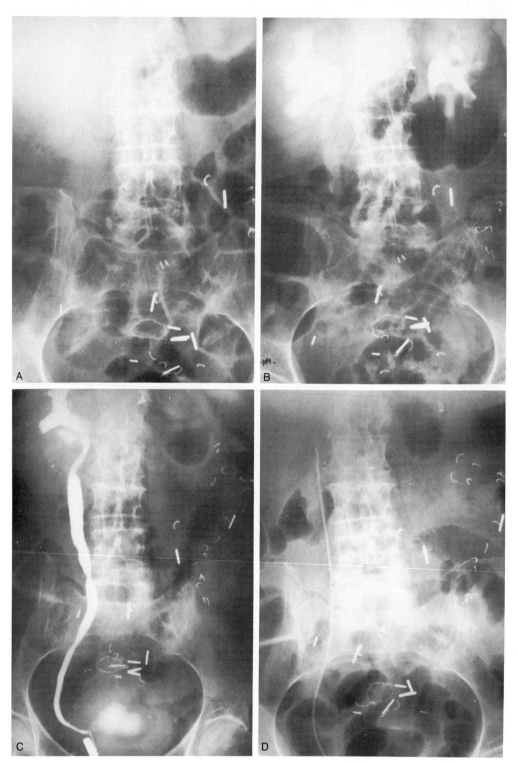

Figure 7–4. A 57-year-old woman who had previously undergone multiple intraabdominal operations presented with severe right flank pain accompanied by a temperature of 103.5°F and shaking chills. A plain abdominal film (A) followed by an excretory urogram (B) were done, which showed obstruction at the mid-portion of the right ureter by a 10 × 12 mm. radiopaque calculus. C, Initially an occlusion tip retrograde ureteropyelogram was performed. This showed slight medial deviation of the mid-ureter and a narrowed region just distal to the site of stone impaction. D, A 6 F spiral tip catheter was passed beyond the calculus, and a brisk flow of cloudy urine was obtained.

Illustration continued on opposite page

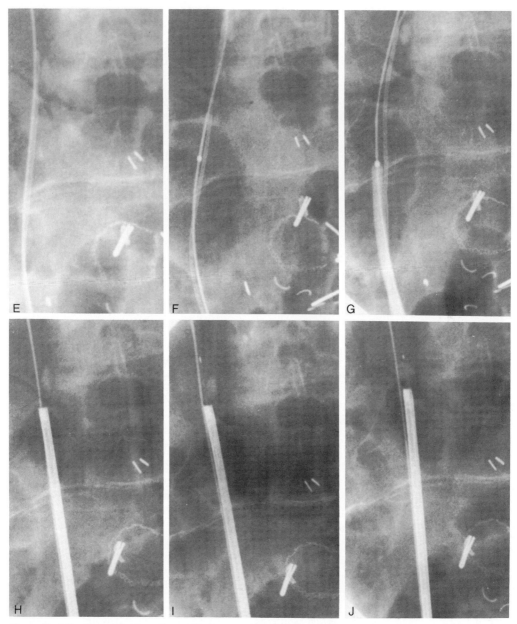

Figure 7–4 Continued E, *Once the patient was stable clinically, endoscopic stone extraction was planned. This radiograph shows the poorly defined calculus near the vertebral body, with the tip of a spiral catheter alongside. A guidewire has also been passed cystoscopically beyond the calculus and is positioned in the renal pelvis. F, A 10 cm. by 5 mm. ureteral balloon dilation catheter was then positioned across the intramural tunnel and lower ureter. This was passed cystoscopically over the previously passed guidewire. G, Inflation of the balloon was carried out, while the maneuver was watched both cystoscopically and fluoroscopically. A 3 ml. syringe was used to inflate the balloon to approximately 100 psi. H, The spiral tip catheter was removed and the operating offset ureteroscope inserted. This radiograph shows the tip of the ureteroscope 1 to 2 cm. distal to the calculus. I, A 3.5 F stone basket is passed through the catheterizing port of the ureteroscope and positioned above the calculus. J, The basket is opened and withdrawn to entrap the stone. This entire process is performed with visual control.*

Illustration continued on following page

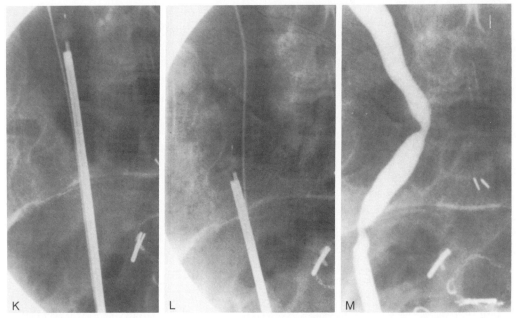

Figure 7—4 Continued K, *This oversized stone could not be extracted intact; therefore, ultrasonic lithotripsy was necessary. Under direct vision, the ultrasonic probe was applied and used to partially fragment the calculus while it was held in position by the basket. L, The calculus could then be pulled partially down the ureter; however, another area of narrowing prohibited passage into the bladder. Therefore, further disintegration was performed at this level. M, The stone was removed and the instrument reinserted to check for any damage to the ureter or any residual stone fragments. A retrograde contrast study was performed. This film demonstrates the area of previous stone impaction in the mid-ureter. A ureteral catheter was left in place for 48 hours.*

is then inserted in place of the telescope and slowly advanced. The position of the probe can be confirmed fluoroscopically, but combined manual control of the stone in the basket and the probe assure the greatest accuracy in localization. Tactile sensation and fluoroscopic visualization assure contact between the probe and stone. The irrigation is then started flowing through the sheath, and suction is applied to the probe.

Table 7—2
TACTILE TECHNIQUE OF URETEROPYELOSCOPIC
ULTRASONIC LITHOTRIPSY

1. Calculus too large to extract through lumen must be disintegrated.
2. Position calculus in basket at tip of ureteropyeloscope.
3. Remove telescope and introduce ultrasound probe.
4. Feel probe against calculus and hear during fragmentation.
5. Apply power when irrigation is running and probe is touching calculus.
6. Confirm position of probe fluoroscopically.
7. Remove ultrasound unit and replace telescope to observe calculus.
8. Repeat steps 2 to 7 as necessary until calculus is small enough to extract safely.
9. Place open-end catheter or diversionary ureteral stent in proper position for post-operative drainage.

The ultrasonic generator foot pedal is then depressed, triggering the disintegration process. Only 10- to 15-second bursts are used after which the telescope is re-inserted to assess progress. Steady pressure is applied to the probe until: (1) the probe moves past the stone (a "give" will be felt), (2) the sound of the probe changes as contact with the calculus is lost; or (3) the end of the 10- to 15-second time period is reached. Often the stone can be removed either completely or partially after one application of the probe. If the stone is still too large to be extracted, further disintegration is required. After a large fragment has been removed, the instrument is re-inserted to the level where the calculus has been lodged to remove other fragments or, if all major fragments have been removed, the procedure is terminated and a ureteral catheter is passed.

Direct Vision Ultrasonic Ureterolithotripsy

Use of the operating ureteropyeloscope with an offset lens permits ureterolithotripsy under direct vision (see Figs. 1–6, 1–10, 1–11, and 1–12).[6] The instruments are of a similar caliber as those of the conventional sheath design but contain an integral telescope with an offset ocular lens, which allows a straight working channel to accommodate a small rigid ultrasound probe. There is also space for a small working device such as a basket or a Fogarty catheter to prevent proximal migration of the calculus. The working channel will accept an instrument no larger than 4 F, but in order to place the ultrasound probe as well, the working instrument must be no more than 3.5 F. Therefore, working capabilities are extremely limited.

Several types of probes are used with the offset system. There are 1.5- and 2.0-mm. probes with hollow cores for aspiration of fragments and irrigation. Also Karl Storz Instruments has developed the TUUL (transurethral ultrasonic lithotriptor) probe which is solid. With this probe, aspiration and irrigation occur through the sheath.

Ureteroscopes are also available with interchangeable lenses, including an offset design telescope that permits placement of an ultrasound probe under direct vision just as with the integral instrument. This design has the specific advantage of accepting standard forward or lateral telescopes in the same sheath (see Figs. 1–10 and 1–11).

Another design has incorporated a fiberoptic bundle for viewing (see Fig. 1–12). The ocular lens is offset from the major axis of the rigid instrument to allow placement of the rigid ultrasound probe under direct vision. Since the ocular lens is flexible, it can be positioned for the operator's convenience. The combination of the small fiberoptic bundle for viewing with an instrument of triangular cross-section provides a relatively larger working channel.

TECHNIQUE

The operating ureteropyeloscope is passed into the urethra, through the bladder, and into the ureter in the same fashion as the conventional sheathed

Table 7–3
DIRECT VISUAL ULTRASONIC URETEROLITHOTRIPSY

1. Visualize calculus ureteroscopically.
2. Engage calculus in basket or obstruct ureter proximally.
3. Impacted calculus may be fragmented in-situ.
4. Apply ultrasound probe to calculus and activate.
5. Continue irrigation with suction through probe.
6. Reposition calculus as necessary.
7. Remove large fragments from ureter.

instrument, since the tip configuration and size are very similar to the standard design (Table 7–3 and Fig. 7–4). As the instrument approaches the calculus, a working instrument can be placed to prevent proximal migration of a stone. A 3.5-F stone basket is then passed under vision, and the calculus is engaged. Alternatively, a balloon catheter such as a 3-F Fogarty can be passed and the balloon inflated proximal to the calculus to prevent migration upward. A basket will hold the stone more firmly than a balloon.

After the calculus has been secured, the ultrasound probe is passed into the working channel of the instrument and applied to the calculus under vision. Irrigation is maintained through the ureteropyeloscope while suction is applied through the ultrasound probe for aspiration of fragments. The probe is repetitively applied to the visible portion of the calculus to fragment it into smaller pieces that can be removed, and the entire calculus can be aspirated if it is sufficiently fragile. Often, removal of irregular extensions of a calculus will permit removal of the entire calculus.

ADVANTAGES

The direct viewing operating ureteropyeloscope appears to be of particular benefit in two circumstances. The impacted ureteral calculus that cannot be bypassed with any working instrument or guidewire may be held securely by the ureter as it is fragmented under vision. Although it is extremely difficult, if not impossible, to fragment such calculi using only tactile or fluoroscopic control with the standard sheathed instrument, the ultrasound probe can be applied to the calculus under direct vision with the operating endoscope. The calculus is then fragmented at the margin either to free it from the ureter or to provide an opening through which a working instrument can be passed to prevent proximal migration.

The operating instrument can also be used to dilate ureteral strictures under vision. The large lumen of the working channel will accept a 5-F balloon dilating catheter, which can be passed into the stricture and inflated under direct vision. Thus, accurate, full dilation of a ureteral narrowing can be assured.

DISADVANTAGES

The offset lens operating ureteropyeloscope presents unique problems from those of the conventional design. If the eyepiece is offset at 45 degrees, the endoscopist's eye is offset from the major axis of the instrument. Thus, the instrument must be advanced at an angle away from the urologist. The position of the endoscope is determined by the position of its tip within the ureter. As an example, the bevel of the tip may pass easily into the ureteral orifice under the overhanging lip of mucosa or it may be turned 180 degrees to allow the bevel to enter the orifice. In each case, the position of the endoscope is determined by the need to position the tip of the instrument within the ureter rather than by the operator's convenience. Thus, at times the offset lens may be placed immediately adjacent to the patient's leg or it may be pointing toward the floor, and the urologist must position his or her head accordingly. These problems have been overcome by instruments with interchangeable lenses and by the combined rigid-flexible design.

The smaller working channel limits the instruments that can be employed under vision. Since the entire sheath is not available at any time because of the integral design of the telescope, only very small fragments of calculi can be withdrawn through the instrument. This small size of the channel also limits the diameter of the ultrasound probe. The smaller probe is less efficient at fragmenting calculi and frequently becomes occluded with fragments. Whenever it is occluded, it must be removed from the instrument and manually cleaned by passing a wire into the lumen of the probe to dislodge the fragment.

PLACEMENT OF A URETERAL CATHETER AT THE END OF THE PROCEDURE

A ureteral catheter should be inserted after every ureteroscopic procedure. Many types of catheters can be used, including standard whistle-tipped catheters, single pigtail diversionary stents, open-end ureteral catheters, and self-retaining internal stents.

One method of catheter insertion is with the ureteroscope still within the ureter. The catheter is passed directly through the sheath and positioned in the renal pelvis.

Fluoroscopy is used or a standard radiograph taken to ensure its proper position. Once the catheter is in place, the ureteroscope is removed, and the catheter is held in position with either another catheter or the obturator of the ureteroscope.

Alternatively, a 0.038-inch guidewire can be left in position and the ureteropyeloscope removed. Cystoscopically or fluoroscopically either an internal ureteral stent or an open-end ureteral catheter is placed over the guidewire and positioned appropriately in the renal pelvis and bladder.

Electrohydraulic Lithotripsy

Another method for fragmentation of oversized calculi is electrohydraulic "shock wave" lithotripsy. This method, using an electrohydraulic shock wave generator and a 3- or 5-F coaxial probe, produces a shock wave that causes cavitation and fragmentation when directed toward a calculus.[7, 8, 9]

The advantages of this method are that standard ureteropyeloscopic sheaths can be used, the procedure is performed under direct visual control, and stone size is effectively reduced to allow subsequent removal or passage of fragments. Since the probe is flexible, it can be passed through a flexible instrument or through the side working channel of a standard ureteroscope or it can be manipulated with a deflecting lever.

The disadvantages include: (1) uncontrolled fragmentation of calculi; there is no provision for removal of small fragments through the probe); (2) a potentially higher incidence of damage to ureteral mucosa; and (3) necessity of a special irrigant (1/6 normal saline). It has been recommended that impacted calculi not be fragmented with this method.[9] However, many urologists have used this technique percutaneously in the ureter for removal of impacted calculi.

TECHNIQUE OF ELECTROHYDRAULIC LITHOTRIPSY

The ureteropyeloscope is inserted into the ureter, and the calculus is approached using the same technique and precautions described previously. Once the calculus is visualized, the coaxial probe is advanced to a point close to the stone but not quite in contact with it. The generator is set on single impulse (not continuous), and the foot pedal is depressed. As the calculus is fragmented, debris may obscure the visual field. It is important to drain the irrigant, to clear the field, and to prevent overheating. Fragmentation is repeated as necessary to reduce the calculus to a size that can be removed.

The Impacted Calculus

A calculus impacted in the ureter presents specific problems for ureteroscopic removal and has proved to be a major obstacle for many urologists learning the techniques of ureteroscopy. Therefore, we have summarized the approach to the impacted calculus.

The firmly impacted calculus may prevent passage of a guidewire or basket or other grasper. Dilation of the ureterovesical junction may then be considerably more difficult. In general, one of the unguided techniques for ureteral dilation should be employed to provide an adequate lumen through the intramural ureter. The techniques and the special problems encountered with the impacted calculus have been discussed in Chapter 5 and earlier in this chapter. As noted, dilation is more difficult if the calculus is located at the level of the ureterovesical junction. When the calculus is located more proximally within the ureter, the guidewire still may be placed far enough into the ureteral lumen for adequate dilation.

After the ureter has been adequately dilated for passage of a ureteroscope, the optimal technique for removal of the stone is to approach it with an operative, direct viewing ureteroscope and then to fragment the calculus in-situ. As the stone is partially fragmented, a guidewire can often be passed beyond the calculus to be left in place as a safety wire. The ureteroscope can then be removed and replaced, leaving the wire within the ureter but still allowing a channel within the instrument for placing a basket.

The calculus can then be fragmented further with the ultrasonic lithotriptor to allow its eventual removal. As long as the calculus remains trapped by the ureteral mucosa, it can be fragmented without placement of a basket, balloon, or other device for holding the calculus. If the stone is dislodged, then it should be held with a basket just as the free-floating stone is restrained.

Occasionally, the calculus can be dislodged with the tip of the ureteroscope and then engaged within a basket. However, if the calculus is located very proximally within the ureter, there is a significant risk of dislodging the calculus into an inaccessible portion of the intrarenal collecting system. Again the preferred technique is to fragment the calculus under direct vision and engage it within a basket as early as possible.

The solid wire probe (TUUL) has also been used under direct vision for the impacted calculus. Although the electrohydraulic lithotripter has been employed for fragmentation of ureteral calculi through the flexible nephroscope in an antegrade fashion, Green and co-workers have recommended against its use for the impacted calculus.[9] They cite the need for flow of irrigant for cooling near the tip of the electrohydraulic probe.

The impacted calculus should not present an insurmountable problem to the urologist. It should be reassuring to the new ureteroscopist to recognize that impacted ureterovesical junction calculi are included in reports of the high success rates seen with distal ureteral calculi.

Proximal Migration of Fragments

One of the major sources of failure in the ureteropyeloscopic removal of calculi has been the proximal migration of fragments into an inaccessible location in the intrarenal collecting system. Despite use of the many techniques described for preventing proximal migration, including limitation of the irrigation pressure, placement of the patient in the reverse Trendelenburg position, and proximal obstruction of the ureter, it may be impossible to prevent migration of all calculi or all fragments. If only tiny fragments of no more than 2 to 3 mm. have migrated, they may be expected to pass spontaneously. However, the entire calculus or larger fragments may not be expected to pass, and they should be retrieved if possible. Often draining irrigant from the ureter will permit the calculus to pass down the ureter to the site where it had been lodged. The attempt to capture it with a basket or other device can then be repeated. Great care should be used to minimize the flow of irrigant, and the patient should be in a steep reverse Trendelenburg position.

Often the fragmented calculus will lodge in the pelvis or a posterior renal calyx and not return immediately to the ureter. The ureteroscope is then passed to the level of the renal pelvis in an attempt to visualize the calculus. Retrieval may be assisted by draining the pelvis in an attempt to bring the calculus to the central portion of the pelvis. Occasionally, it is possible to pass a stone basket into the pelvis, open it widely, and force the

Table 7–4

SUCCESS RATE OF URETEROPYELOSCOPIC STONE REMOVAL

Author	No. of Patients	Percentage of Stones Removed
Lyon et al[10]	133	78
Sosa et al[11]	46	78
Khuri et al[12]	43	84
Green and Lytton[9]	36	82
Bagley et al[13]	70	87
Epple and Reuter[14]	154	57
Ghoniem and El-Kappany[15]	64	89
Kahn[16]	120	95
Keating et al[17]	51	69

calculus into the basket by draining the pelvis. If the calculus is located laterally within the pelvis, it may be necessary to use the lateral viewing telescope. Then one of the deflecting baskets or graspers can be passed to retrieve the calculus. If a flexible ureteroscope is available, that may be helpful in viewing the calculus and positioning an instrument to retrieve it.

If an extracorporeal shock wave lithotripter is available, it may be preferable to place a self-retaining ureteral stent to obstruct passage of the calculus back into the ureter and discontinue the procedure. Then in a second procedure, the patient can be treated with the ESWL with an expectation of success, since a small ureteral calculus is then positioned more favorably within the larger intrarenal collecting system.

Results

The reported success rates for ureteropyeloscopic stone retrieval are listed in Table 7–4. These results represent the initial work of many pioneers in the field. Not every endoscopist reported the failure rate according to stone position; however, our results show the expected high rate of success in removing distal and mid-ureteral stones and the relatively poor results in removing renal pelvic stones (Table 7–5).

The overall success rate for stone removal from the ureter is approximately 80 per cent.[6] As expected, most success has been enjoyed for stones

Table 7–5

URETEROPYELOSCOPIC STONE REMOVAL BY LOCATION
(percentage removed)

Location	Author						
	Lyon et al[10]	Sosa et al[11]	Khuri et al[12]	Green and Lytton[9]	Bagley et al[13]	Kahn[16]	Keating et al[17]
Upper Ureter	50	33	50	22	60	—	58
Mid-Ureter	83	66	80	75	67	71	36
Lower Ureter	96	90	95	94	97	99	84

in the lower ureter, where over 90 per cent of attempts have been successful. In the mid-third of the ureter, 60–80 per cent of the stones have been removed. The combined success rate for stone removal in the lower two thirds of the ureter is 80 per cent. In the proximal ureter and renal pelvis, only one half of stones are extracted. In contrast, success rates of over 90 per cent are reported for stone extraction from the proximal ureter by percutaneous nephrostolithotomy. Extracorporeal shock wave lithotripsy is currently being investigated for its efficacy in renal and proximal ureteral calculi and, thus far, results are very encouraging. At the present time, it appears that the extraction of oversized calculi from the lower two thirds of the ureter, including impacted calculi, is the main indication for ureteropyeloscopy in stone disease.

References

1. Huffman JL, Bagley DH, and Lyon ES: Treatment of distal ureteral calculi using a rigid ureteroscope. Urology 20:574, 1982.
2. Das S: Transurethral ureteroscopy and stone manipulation under direct vision. J Urol 125:112, 1981.
3. Ford TE, Watson GM, and Wickham JEA: Transurethral ureteroscopic retrieval of ureteric stones. Br J Urol 55:626, 1983.
4. Huffman JL, Bagley DH, Schoenberg HW, and Lyon ES: Transurethral removal of large ureteral and renal pelvic calculi using ureteroscopic ultrasonic lithotripsy. J Urol 130:31, 1983.
5. Howards SS, Merrill E, Harris S, and Cohen J: Ultrasonic lithotripsy—laboratory evaluation. Invest Urol 11:273, 1974.
6. Huffman JL, Bagley DH, and Lyon ES: Transurethral ureteropyeloscopy. In Bagley DH, Huffman JL, and Lyon ES (eds.): *Urologic Endoscopy: A Manual and Atlas*. Boston, Little Brown and Company, 1985, pp. 185–206.
7. Rouvalis P: Electronic lithotripsy for vesical calculus with "Urat 1." An experience of 100 cases and an experimental application of the method to stones in the upper urinary tract. Br J Urol 42:486, 1970.
8. Raney AM and Handler J: Electrohydraulic nephrolithotripsy. Urology 6:439, 1975.
9. Green DF and Lytton B: Early experience with electrohydraulic lithotripsy of ureteral calculi using direct vision ureteroscopy. J Urol 133:767, 1985.
10. Lyon ES, Bagley DH, and Huffman JL: Ureteropyeloscopic diagnosis and removal of ureteral and renal pelvic calculi. Presented at Third Congress of the International Society of Urologic Endoscopy, Karlsruhe, Federal Republic of Germany, August, 1984.
11. Sosa RE, Huffman JL, Riehle RA, and Vaughan ED: Ureteropyeloscopy: Pitfalls and early complications of ureteral stone extraction. Presented at XXth Congess Société Internationale d'Urologie. Vienna, June, 1985.
12. Khuri FJ, Peartree RJ, Ruotolo RA, and Valvo JR: Rigid ureteropyeloscopy. NY State J Med 85:205, 1985.
13. Bagley DH, Seeger R, and Rittenberg MH: Ureteropyeloscopic removal of ureteral calculi (unpublished data).
14. Epple W and Reuter H: Ureterorenoscopy for diagnosis and therapy. Presented at XXth Congress Société Internationale d'Urologie. Vienna, June, 1985.
15. Ghoniem MA and El-Kappany HA: Ureteroscopy for the treatment of ureteral calculi. Presented at XXth Congress S.I.U. Vienna, June, 1985.
16. Kahn RI: Endourological treatment of ureteral calculi. J Urol 135:239, 1986.
17. Keating MA, Heney NM, Young HH, Kerr WS Jr., O'Leary MP, and Dretler SP: Ureteroscopy: The initial experience. J Urol 135:689, 1986.

CHAPTER 8

Diagnostic and Therapeutic Approaches to Upper Tract Urothelial Tumors

JEFFRY L. HUFFMAN

Primary epithelial tumors of the upper urinary tract often pose a formidable diagnostic challenge and a therapeutic dilemma. An important consideration in managing patients thought to have upper tract malignancies is the identification of the patients who might benefit from a conservative or renal unit–sparing approach. Since pre-operative clinical staging methods for upper tract tumors have been inconsistent and fairly unreliable, therapeutic guidelines have been drawn mainly from retrospective analyses of various surgical approaches or from pathologic mapping studies of nephroureterectomy specimens.

Albarran in 1902 may have made the first endoscopic diagnosis of an upper tract tumor when he discovered a tumor protruding from a ureteral orifice at cystoscopy.[1] Although information regarding treatment of bladder tumors has made great strides over the intervening years, largely because of endoscopic clinical staging techniques, relatively little information has been gained in the approach to upper tract urothelial tumors.

However, the recent advance in the design of endoscopic instrumentation, especially the rigid ureteropyeloscope, has potentially opened the ureter and renal pelvis to routine endoscopic assessment. Although no categorical answer to the question of which patients can be treated conservatively can be made at this time, the urologist can obtain much more information pre-operatively in regard to tumor grade, site, multicentricity, and stage.

We have found the ureteropyeloscope to have uses very similar to those of the cystoscope. These include: diagnosis of upper urinary tract tumors, surveillance of the urothelium following previous therapy, and occasionally primary endoscopic treatment of selected tumors.[2]

Flexible ureteropyeloscopes complement the rigid instrument since they often are able to be passed through a tortuous ureter and into the intrarenal collecting system for diagnosis. They are limited, however, in their capability for obtaining biopsy specimens.

Diagnosis of Upper Tract Urothelial Tumors

The diagnosis of upper tract tumors rests upon endoscopic identification of the lesion and histologic examination of biopsy material. Most often filling defects are recognized easily, and the differentiation among tumor, blood clot, uric acid calculus, and sloughed papilla can be made by endoscopic appearance alone (Table 8–1).[3]

Table 8–1
INITIAL PRESENTATION OF PATIENTS EVALUATED
URETEROSCOPICALLY

Indication	No. of Patients	Tumor Identified
Filling defect	30	19
Obstruction	5	2
Tumor at orifice	10	6
Hematuria only	11	0
Abnormal cytology only	3	0
Total	59	27

PAPILLARY UROTHELIAL TUMORS

Papillary tumors are the most common types of tumors identified in the upper urinary tract. The papillomas and the better differentiated transitional cell carcinoma have a typical papillary frond appearance, with finger-like projections and a central fibrovascular core. The less differentiated tumors are more solid appearing, possibly with areas of necrosis, calcification, and ulceration. The differential diagnosis includes benign ureteral polyps, ureteritis cystica, and ureteritis follicularis.

NON-PAPILLARY CARCINOMA-IN-SITU

Non-papillary carcinoma-in-situ (CIS) is recognized as a velvety red, slightly raised region of the ureteral mucosa. Similar to its identification within the bladder, it is most easily seen during the initial pass of the instrument and with the ureter only partially distended. Once the mucosa has been traumatized by the instrument, endoscopic visualization of flat CIS may be impossible.

INFLAMMATORY POLYPS

Inflammatory polyps may be very difficult to differentiate from papillary tumors; biopsy and microscopic examination are often required to make a diagnosis. They are most commonly seen in conjunction with ureteral stones, indwelling ureteral catheters, or urinary tract infection. Besides the association with the above findings, another endoscopic clue to the benign nature of an inflammatory polyp is the vascular pattern. Unlike papillary tumors, which have a central fibrovascular core, inflammatory polyps will exhibit a peripheral or spheroid vascular pattern.

URIC ACID CALCULUS

Uric acid calculi are extremely hard stones that are usually easily recognizable. Unlike calcium oxalate stones, which have a very crystalline structure, urate stones are smooth and rounded with a characteristic orange-

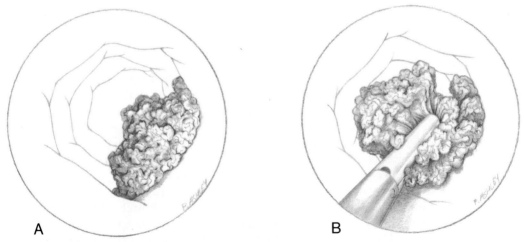

Figure 8–1. *When a ureteral lesion is identified ureteroscopically, biopsy is performed during the initial pass of the instrument. The flexible cup forceps is extended from the sheath and opened parallel to the ureteral wall (A). Once the tissue is within the jaws, the forceps is closed and gently pulled from the ureter (B).*

red color. The differential diagnosis includes blood clots; however, blood clots fragment easily when probed with a catheter or the ureteroscope sheath.

Biopsy

The biopsy of abnormalities within the ureter or pelvis is at first very awkward for the endoscopist. This is because of the relation of the instrument and forceps to the location of the tumors. In the bladder (a spherical structure), the forceps can be applied perpendicular to the area from which the biopsy material is to be taken. However, in the ureter (a tubular structure) the forceps must be applied parallel to the ureteral mucosa.

Biopsy is performed during the initial pass of the ureteroscope. If an attempt is made to examine the entire upper tract and then remove a specimen for biopsy, the lesion may be inadvertently traumatized or avulsed during instrument passage. When the lesion is identified, the 5 F (1.6 mm. diameter) cup forceps is carefully advanced with its jaws parallel to the ureteral wall (Fig. 8–1). The intraluminal portion of the lesion is then grasped with the jaws and pulled free from the ureter using gentle traction on the forceps.

The size of the biopsy specimen obtained is minute and should be placed in preservative at once. Special notation is made so that the pathology department is aware of the small size of the specimen.

One problem occasionally encountered is that the biopsy specimen is lost as it is pulled through the instrument sheath. To avoid this problem, either remove the telescope, thus providing more room within the sheath, or remove the entire ureteroscope including the forceps.

Resection and Fulguration

The technique of ureteroscopic resection is very similar to that of pediatric resection using a pediatric resectoscope. The instrumentation, illustrated in Chapter 1, is also very similar to pediatric resectoscopes except for its added length. The very fine construction of the resectoscope loops provides excellent control over depth and location of resection.

Basic transurethral electrosurgery principles are maintained. A non-conducting irrigant such as glycine or water should be used, and the use of the appropriate setting on the coagulation and cutting currents provides the most effective surgery with the least tissue injury.

The actual mechanics of resecting an upper urinary tract tumor are different from those used in the bladder or prostate. Only intraluminal tumor is resected, and no attempt is made to take deep arcing bites into the ureteral wall. For this reason, the tip of the resectoscope is positioned directly distal to the tumor (Fig. 8–2). The loop is extended beyond the tumor, and prior to activating the power, the tissue is drawn back toward the tip of the instrument. When the tissue is either inside the insulation or directly outside it, the power is started and the tissue resected. This method helps ensure that only the desired tissue is cut and prevents injury to the surrounding ureteral wall.

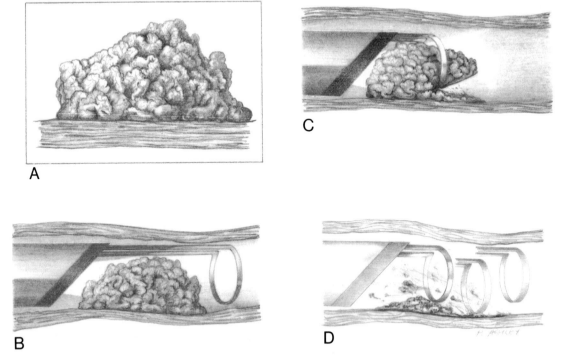

Figure 8–2. Ureteroscopic resection of a tumor (A). The instrument is positioned immediately distal to the lesion, and the resectoscope loop is extended past the tumor (B). Prior to activating the cutting power, the tissue is drawn into the sheath, thus minimizing the chance of ureteral injury (C). The base of the tumor and any bleeding sites can be lightly fulgurated (D).

Table 8–2
SUCCESS RATE IN PERFORMING URETEROSCOPIC PROCEDURES

Result	No. of Patients	Percentage
Completed satisfactorily	54	92
Unsuccessful	5	8
Total	59	100

Following resection of all intraluminal tumor, the base of the lesion is lightly fulgurated with the resectoscope loop. Smooth to-and-fro movements are used to cauterize the region of the resected tumor lightly, and only the power needed to cause fulguration is used.

Fulguration is also possible with a Bugbee electrode. The 5 F probe is advanced through the sheath and gently positioned on the area to be fulgurated. With irrigation flowing, the coagulation current is activated. Irrigation is necessary to maintain clear visualization and to dissipate the bubbles that are produced.

Results

In the period from 1977 to 1984, 59 patients were evaluated ureteroscopically at the University of Chicago Hospital and Clinics (24) and at Memorial Sloan-Kettering Cancer Center (35).[4, 5] These patients presented with findings suggestive of an upper tract urothelial tumor including: filling defects, hematuria, tumor near or within the ureteral orifice in the bladder, obstruction, and positive results of cytologic studies (Table 8–1).

The ureteroscopic procedure was completed successfully in 54 patients (90%) and had to be aborted in five patients (Table 8–2). Two of the failures were due to an inability to dilate the orifice, one failure was because of an inability to insert the instrument, and two were because of an inability to reach the level of the lesion within the renal pelvis. In the two patients in whom the orifice could not be dilated, the procedures were attempted prior to the routine use of guidewire methods of dilation, and most likely could have been completed with the instrumentation currently available. The patient in whom the instrument could not be inserted had a very delicate ureter that would not distend at any level to accommodate the instrument. Another patient had a very narrow proximal ureter which could not be traversed even after dilation. The final patient had a crossed-fused, ectopic ureter (see Fig. 6–5). Although the ureteroscope could be passed to the level of the proximal ureter, it was not possible to enter the renal pelvis.

The findings in the 54 patients successfully evaluated are listed in Table 8–3. Twenty-seven urothelial tumors, one metastatic squamous cell carcinoma, and three uric acid calculi were diagnosed; one patient had bleeding localized to the lower pole infundibulum of the kidney, and 22 patients had no abnormality detected.

Of the 27 patients with urothelial tumors, six subsequently underwent nephroureterectomy, three segmental ureterectomy, 16 primary ureteroscopic fulguration or resection, and two patients who had metastatic cancer

Table 8–3
URETEROSCOPIC FINDINGS

Finding		No. of Patients
Urothelial tumor		27
Metastatic tumor		1
Uric acid stone		3
Bleeding, localized		1
No abnormality		22
	Total	54

underwent systemic chemotherapy (Table 8–4). The results from patients who underwent nephroureterectomy enabled correlation of the clinical ureteroscopic staging (T-stage) with that obtained by pathologic mapping (P-stage) (Table 8–5). Patients number 3 and 5 were correctly staged clinically; however, patients 1, 2, 4, and 6 were all understaged clinically with ureteroscopic mapping. This finding is not surprising with these patients, since each had extensive tumors involving the pelvis and calyces.

Patient number 5 presented with total, gross, painless hematuria, and excretory urography revealed a 2-cm. filling defect in the renal pelvis. Ureteroscopy was performed, and the biopsy specimen confirmed a papilloma (Fig. 8–3). A nephroureterectomy was then performed, and the entire ureter and intrarenal collecting system were mapped pathologically (Fig. 8–4). In this instance appropriate staging was achieved by the ureteroscopic procedure.

Three patients underwent segmental ureterectomy and then were evaluated ureteroscopically as a surveillance procedure (Table 8–6). All tumors were accurately staged pre-operatively and each had identical T- and P-stages. Patient number 1 has subsequently undergone eight follow up surveillance procedures. Three low-grade recurrences were identified asynchronously at or near the region of the anastomosis. These were all fulgurated, and thus far the patient has had no evidence of metastatic spread of the cancer or diminished renal function. Patients number 2 and 3 underwent segmental ureterectomies for mid-ureteral papillomas. There was no endoscopic evidence of multicentricity of the tumors at the time of the initial diagnostic procedure. Thus far, one follow up procedure that showed no tumor recurrence has been performed on each of these patients.

Sixteen patients had apparently localized, low-grade appearing tumors identified ureteroscopically (Tables 8–7 and 8–8). Following biopsy, these patients were all treated primarily by ureteroscopic resection or fulguration.

Table 8–4
INITIAL TREATMENT FOLLOWING DIAGNOSIS

Treatment		No. of Patients
Nephroureterectomy		6
Segmental ureterectomy		3
Systemic chemotherapy		2
Ureteroscopic resection or fulguration		16
	Total	27

Table 8–5
CORRELATION OF URETEROSCOPIC BIOPSY STAGING WITH
PATHOLOGIC STAGING AFTER NEPHROURETERECTOMY*

Patient No.	Ureteroscopic Biopsy	Pathologic Staging	Tumor Site
1	Grade III	Grade III and CIS	pelvis/calyx
2	Grade III	Grade III-P2	pelvis
3	papilloma	papilloma	mid-ureter
4	papilloma	Grade II-P2 and CIS	pelvis/calyx
5	papilloma and CIS	papilloma and CIS	pelvis
6	Grade II-T2	Grade III-P3	mid-ureter

*CIS = carcinoma in-situ; T2 and P2 = tumors extend into muscularis mucosa; P3 = tumors extend into peri-ureteral tissue.

Follow up was then done at two- to three-month intervals (Table 8–9). Thus far a total of 47 surveillance procedures have been performed in these patients. With an average follow up of 16 months, biopsy and fulguration have been done on 14 low-grade recurrences in five patients. One patient (number 2) died of a myocardial infarction; however, the remaining 15 patients are alive and have no apparent evidence of dissemination of their tumors.

Discussion

Many unanswered questions exist as to the role of ureteroscopy in the management of upper tract urothelial tumors. Certainly its value in diagnosis

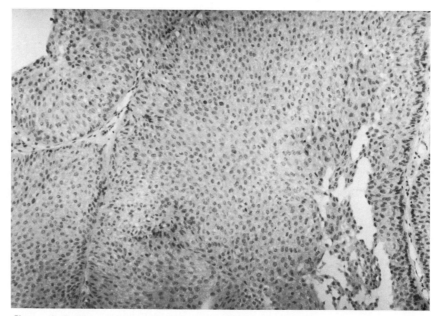

Figure 8–3. This ureteroscopy biopsy specimen of a renal pelvic papilloma shows essentially normal urothelium by cytologic features arranged in a papillary pattern (magnification, 10×).

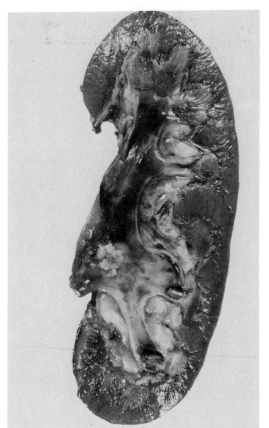

Figure 8–4. Following nephroureterectomy, the entire kidney and ureter were mapped pathologically. This is a hemisection of the kidney prior to sectioning, revealing the papillary tumor on the anterior renal pelvic walls.

Table 8–6
RESULTS OF SURVEILLANCE PROCEDURES FOLLOWING SEGMENTAL URETERECTOMY

Patient No.	No. of Follow Up Procedures	Follow Up (mos.)	No. of Recurrences
1	8	36	4 (papilloma and Grade I)
2	1	6	0
3	0	2	0

Table 8–7
INITIAL TUMOR GRADE IN PATIENTS TREATED PRIMARILY BY
URETEROSCOPY*

Tumor	No. of Patients
Papilloma	8
Papillary CIS†	1
Grade I TCC†	5
Grade II TCC	1
Grade III TCC	1
Total	16

*Staging from Koss LG: Tumors of the urinary bladder. Atlas of Tumor Pathology, Armed Forces Institute of Pathology, 1975, second series, fascicle 2, pp 19–51.
†CIS = carcinoma-in-situ; TCC = transitional cell carcinoma.

Table 8–8
TUMOR SITE IN PATIENTS TREATED PRIMARILY BY
URETEROSCOPY

Site	No. of Patients
Lower ureter	13
Upper ureter	0
Renal pelvis	3
Total	16

Table 8–9
RESULTS OF SURVEILLANCE PROCEDURES FOLLOWING
PRIMARY URETEROSCOPIC TREATMENT*

Patient No.	No. of Follow Up Procedures	Follow Up (mos.)	No. of Recurrences (Grade)
1	14	75	6 (papillomas-fulg.)
2	13	48	2 (papillomas-fulg.)
3	5	16	4 (Grade I-fulg.)
4	2	16	0
5	3	12	0
6	3	11	1 (CIS-fulg.)
7	could not perform follow up procedure		
8	2	8	0
9	2	9	1 (CIS-fulg.)
10	1	7	0
11	1	6	0
12	1	6	0
13	0	3	0
14	0	3	0
15	0	1	0
16	0	1	0

*Fulg. = Fulguration; CIS = carcinoma-in-situ.

is obvious. This includes the initial evaluation of patients with upper tract abnormalities and the surveillance of patients who have previously undergone segmental resections. Its role as a therapeutic modality needs much more investigation. The most critical question is the accuracy of endoscopic staging, and thus far this appears good for ureteral tumors but poor for renal pelvic tumors.

Identifying the tumors endoscopically not only allows thorough mapping of the urothelium but also allows tissue to be obtained by a closed route. The potential importance of closed biopsy is illustrated in a report from the Mayo Clinic in which three patients suffered the recurrence of transitional cell tumor in the renal fossa following open pyeloscopic biopsy and subsequent nephroureterectomy.[6]

The ability to map the urothelium gives the urologist much more clinical confidence when planning a segmental ureterectomy. The extent of tumor involvement is determined pre-operatively and a clear margin of resection is assured.

Case Examples

PATIENT NO. 1

A 53-year-old white man presented with an acute onset of total gross painless hematuria. He had undergone a left radical nephrectomy for renal cell carcinoma four years prior to this presentation. Excretory urography showed a solitary right kidney with normal function but with a renal pelvic filling defect (Fig. 8–5). Cystoscopy and retrograde pyelography confirmed the renal pelvic filling defect, and the patient was referred for a ureteroscopic evaluation. He was otherwise in excellent medical condition. The patient underwent cystoscopy, a retrograde pyelogram, and ureteroscopic visualization of the renal pelvis. A stalk-like papillary tumor was seen arising from the middle portion of the right kidney and extending to the region of the ureteral pelvic junction. Using the ureteroscopic resectoscope, this lesion was partially resected at the time of the first procedure. Pathologic review of the specimen revealed pure papilloma. There were no other tumors seen within the renal pelvis or ureter. The patient was reexamined four weeks later, and at that time the flexible biopsy forceps was used to remove the remainder of the papillary tumor. A Bugbee electrode was used to cauterize the base. The patient has been followed for fifteen months. The retrograde study shows no filling defects, and endoscopically he has been free of disease with negative urinary cytology.

PATIENT NO. 2

A 51-year-old patient had a history of recurrent (low grade and low stage) bladder cancer. However, on a routine excretory urographic examination, a distal ureteral filling defect was identified (Fig. 8–6). He was treated by nephroureterectomy, and the tumor was found to be a superficial

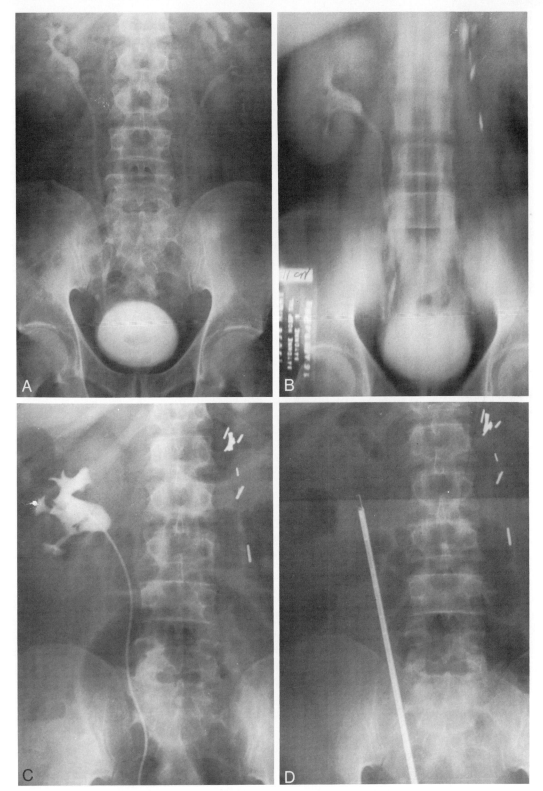

Figure 8–5. A, *This excretory urogram was performed in a 53-year-old man with total gross painless hematuria. He was found to have a left renal mass, and a left radical nephrectomy was performed. Pathologically, a stage I renal carcinoma was found.* B, *Four years after the initial procedure, the patient again developed hematuria. Excretory urography revealed a questionable right renal pelvic filling defect. Urinary cytology was negative.* C, *A contrast study performed through a ureteral catheter confirmed the filling defect, and ureteropyeloscopy with biopsy revealed a localized papilloma.* D, *The ureteroscopic resectoscope was inserted, and the tumor was partially resected. The remainder of the tumor was removed by biospy forceps and the base fulgurated with a Bugbee electrode.*

Illustration continued on following page

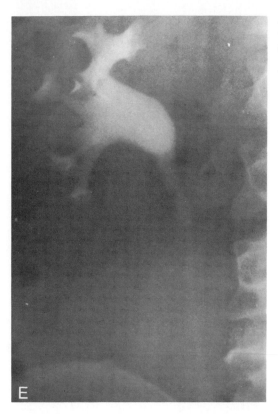

Figure 8–5 Continued E, *An excretory urogram was done 15 months after the procedure and revealed prompt function with no evidence of recurrent tumor. The patient was asymptomatic clinically and endoscopically and continued to have negative urinary cytology.*

grade II carcinoma. Multiple transurethral bladder resections were undertaken over the next two to three years. However, the patient developed worsening hydroureteronephrosis in his remaining left kidney, and on cystoscopic examination tumor was seen to exit the left ureteral orifice. A distal ureterectomy and reimplant was performed; the patient was again found to have a non-invasive grade II carcinoma of the distal ureter on review of the specimen. The patient did well for twelve months. However, he again developed positive urinary cytology. Ureteroscopy revealed five separate papillary tumors in his remaining left kidney. Using the ureteroscopic resectoscope, these tumors were resected completely. All tumor was found to be grade II, with some tumor invading the lamina propria. Since the patient had vesicoureteral reflux, he was treated with topical BCG in the bladder. His endoscopic examination three months following the ureteroscopic resection showed a pristine ureter and no evidence of urothelial abnormality. He will also be followed at routine three-month intervals.

PATIENT NO. 3

A 42-year-old woman with a history of carcinoma of the cervix presented with gross painless hematuria. The excretory urogram (Fig. 8–7) revealed left hydronephrosis with poor visualization of the mid-left ureter. On cystoscopic examination, the bleeding was found to be localized to the left

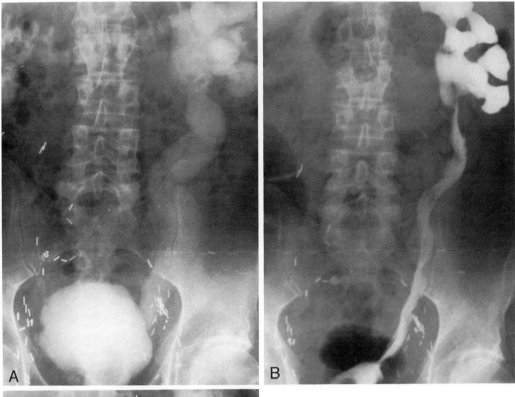

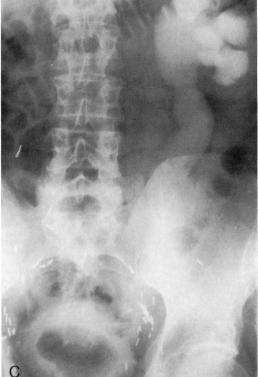

Figure 8–6. A, A 51-year-old man had previously undergone a right nephroureterectomy for a localized distal ureteral carcinoma. He then was found on cystoscopic examination to have a tumor from the left ureteral orifice. A distal left ureterectomy with implant was done. One year later the patient developed positive urinary cytology. A cystogram (shown above) revealed free reflux and several possible filling defects. B, Ureteroscopy was performed and five separate papillary tumors were identified. These were all resected and were found to be noninvasive grade II urothelial carcinomas. This catheter injection study done 24 hours postoperatively revealed no obstruction or extravasation. C, The patient then underwent a 6-week induction course of intravesical BCG. Three months later, this excretory urogram showed stable renal function. The patient was endoscopically free of disease, had negative urinary cytology, and had a normal serum creatinine level.

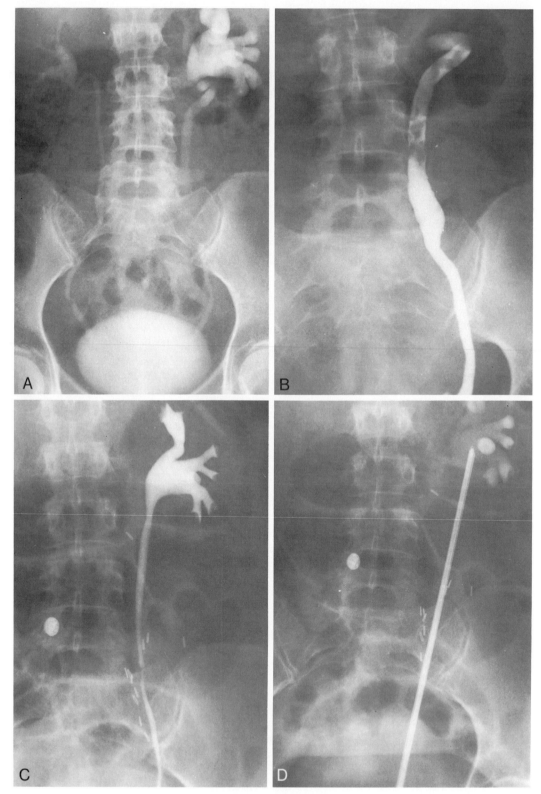

Figure 8–7. See legend on opposite page.

collecting system, and a retrograde pyelogram revealed a mid-ureteral filling defect with evidence of a blood clot proximally. Under ureteroscopic control, a biopsy specimen of the filling defect was obtained; a papilloma was diagnosed, and the surrounding urothelium was normal by observation and biopsy. A segmented ureterectomy was performed. Pathologically, the lesion was confirmed to be a papilloma. Two months later a retrograde pyelogram showed an irregular lumen near the anastomatic site. Surveillance ureteroscopy was performed and a normal ureter was found, without evidence of tumor recurrence. The patient has now been followed for eighteen months and has remained disease-free.

References

1. Whitmore WF Jr.: Management of urothelial tumors of the upper collecting system. In Skinner DG (Ed.): *Urological Cancer*. New York, Grune & Stratton, 1983, pp. 181–198.
2. Huffman JL, Bagley DH, and Lyon ES: Extending cystoscopic techniques into the ureter and renal pelvis—Experience with ureteroscopy and pyeloscopy. JAMA 250:2004–2008, 1983.
3. Huffman JL, Bagley DH, and Lyon ES: Abnormal ureter and renal pelvis. In Bagley DH, Huffman JL, and Lyon ES (Eds.): Urologic Endoscopy—*A Manual and Atlas*. Boston, Little, Brown & Co., 1984, pp. 80–88.
4. Huffman JL, Morse MJ, Bagley DH, Herr HW, Lyon ES, and Whitmore WF Jr.: Endoscopic diagnosis and treatment of upper tract urothelial tumors. Cancer 55:1422–1428, 1985.
5. Huffman JL: Ureteropyeloscopic approach to upper tract urothelial tumors. World J Urol 3:58–63, 1985.
6. Tomera KM, Leary FJ, and Zincke H: Pyeloscopy in urothelial tumors. J Urol 127:1088–1089, 1982.

Figure 8–7. A, A 42-year-old woman with a history of carcinoma of the cervix presented with gross painless hematuria. An excretory urogram revealed left hydronephrosis. B, Cystoscopically, bleeding was localized to the left ureteral orifice, and a retrograde ureterogram revealed a mid-ureteral filling defect with evidence of a blood clot above. C, On ureteroscopic examination, the lesion was identified as a localized papillary tumor. Biopsy proved this to be a papilloma. A segmental ureterectomy was performed. This retrograde ureterogram was performed 3 months after the initial surgical procedure and showed several irregularities near the anastomotic site. D, Surveillance ureteroscopy was done, and no abnormalities were identified. The patient has been followed with endoscopic examination for 18 months and no recurrences have been identified.

CHAPTER 9

Post-Operative Care of the Patient

JEFFRY L. HUFFMAN
DEMETRIUS H. BAGLEY

The patient who has undergone a ureteroscopic procedure does not require specific attention different than that for patients who have undergone transurethral surgery within the bladder. Similar to the immediate post-operative care after routine transurethral resection of the prostate or bladder, care of the ureteroscopic patient involves basic monitoring of temperature, urine output, and pain. This enables rapid recognition of problems, including bacteremia, ureteral obstruction, or urinary extravasation, should they develop.

Long-term follow up includes surveillance of the structural and functional integrity of the urinary tract. Our experience has shown these procedures to be relatively innocuous as compared with open surgery on the upper urinary tract, which may, in part, be due to the close monitoring performed on these patients.

Immediate Post-Operative Care

The goal of care in the immediate post-operative period is to allow quick recovery from the procedure and prompt discharge from the hospital at full working capacity. The most important aspect of this is the early recognition and quick correction of complications should they occur. This involves maintaining certain routine post-operative measures and instructing the nursing staff on the care of these patients and the recognition of abnormalities.

A list of typical routine post-operative orders is given in Table 9–1. Vital signs are measured in the recovery room every 15 minutes until the patient is awake and alert, then they are taken every 4 hours. Special attention is paid to the possible development of sepsis, which would be indicated in part by tachycardia and fever and possibly hypotension in the later stages.

There are no restrictions placed upon the patient's activity as long as he or she is awake and alert. Certainly, precautions should be taken with patients with indwelling catheters to ensure that catheters do not become dislodged when the patient ambulates.

Immediately following the procedure, when the patients are alert, they are allowed to take liquids by mouth. The diet is then advanced liberally as long as there is no nausea, vomiting, or abdominal distention.

Urine output is closely monitored in every patient. If there is a sudden

Table 9–1
ROUTINE POST-URETEROSCOPY ORDERS (70 kg. adult)

1. Vital signs: Q15 minutes until stable, then Q4 hours.
2. Activity: Ambulate as tolerated when alert.
3. Diet: Clear liquids, advance to regular diet as tolerated.
4. Attach ureteral and Foley catheters to separate drainage.
5. Record separate urinary outputs. Notify urologist if output from either catheter decreases markedly.
6. IV fluids: D5/0.45% normal saline at 125 ml./hour.
7. Cefazolin 1 gm. IVPB Q6 hours (in patients with infected urine or in patients who have had calculi removed).
8. Morphine sulfate 8 to 10 mg. IM Q4 hours prn.
9. Acetaminophen #3, 1 po Q4 hours prn.

Note: Underlying medical illnesses or previous medication allergies will alter the above general guidelines.

decrease in output from either the Foley catheter or the ureteral catheter, the nursing staff should immediately notify the urologist. The etiology of the decreased urine output must then be determined. This will be discussed in greater detail in a subsequent section.

PERI-OPERATIVE ANTIBIOTICS

In our early experience with ureteropyeloscopy we encountered a patient who developed acute pyelonephritis following a diagnostic procedure performed for evaluation of a filling defect in the renal pelvis. (The defect was found to be a uric acid calculus.) Although the preoperative urine culture was sterile and the patient had no signs or symptoms of urinary infection prior to the procedure, 6 hours after the procedure she developed a fever of 38.5°C and shaking chills. An excretory urogram was done at the time of the septic episode, and it showed no obstruction or extravasation. The patient was treated with broad spectrum antibiotics initially (an aminoglycoside plus ampicillin) and became afebrile within 48 hours. In retrospect, there was a positive blood culture for *Proteus mirabilis* and the same organism grew in the urine culture.

This patient's episode plus the high possibility of contamination during these sometimes long and complicated procedures and of pyelovenous backflow has led us to consider the use of antibiotics routinely, when approaching upper tract calculi, immediately before the procedure and for 24 hours after the procedure. Certainly, if a preoperative urine culture is positive or if the patient exhibits signs of or gives symptoms of urinary tract infection prior to the scheduled procedure, he or she is treated with parenteral antibiotics for 24 hours preoperatively. We do not routinely use antibiotics when evaluating upper tract tumors unless a urine culture or urinalysis suggests infection.

ANALGESICS

The dilation of the ureteral orifice and intramural ureter to 15 F is accompanied by pain. This is one of the reasons ureteroscopic procedures are performed under general anesthesia. Dilation to this level would be intolerable for most patients when awake.

Post-operatively, patients frequently complain of lower quadrant discomfort on the ipsilateral side of the ureteroscopic procedure, which is thought to be secondary to the dilation of the ureter. Occasionally, this pain does require parenteral analgesics, but their use is usually limited to the first 24 hours following the procedure.

Many patients examined early in our experience complained of flank pain post-operatively without evidence of ureteral obstruction or pyelonephritis. This was thought to be secondary to overdistension of the collecting system, since during the procedure irrigating fluid pressure is directly applied to the intrarenal collection system. Simply by maintaining a lower level of irrigating pressure (less than 30 cm.), we were able to eliminate this complaint.

If flank pain is elicited following a procedure, analgesics are necessary. In these instances, however, it is mandatory that other etiologies for the pain other than overdistension be excluded, such as ureteral obstruction, pyelonephritis, or urinary extravasation (Table 9–2).

URETERAL CATHETER OR STENT

Indwelling ureteral catheters are employed following ureteroscopic surgery, generally in conjunction with a Foley catheter. The use of catheters is necessary in any type of ureteroscopic procedure, but it is especially important when upper urinary tract calculi are extracted or upper tract tumors are fulgurated or resected. The purpose of the routine use of catheters is twofold: diversion of urine while the urothelium heals and drainage of urine in case edematous obstruction exists.

A very important part of the post-operative monitoring of the patient is following the urinary output from these catheters. Certainly, a sudden decrease in the amount of drainage from the ureteral catheter implies obstruction of the catheter, displacement of the catheter, or proximal urinary extravasation. For these reasons separate drainage devices are used for the ureteral catheter and the Foley catheter, with each volume recorded separately by the nursing staff.

Table 9–2
POSSIBLE PROBLEMS IN THE IMMEDIATE POST-OPERATIVE PERIOD

Problem	Findings	Diagnosis	Treatment
Pyelonephritis	Fever Flank pain	Panculture IVP or ultrasound	Appropriate antibiotics
Ureteral obstruction	Fever Flank pain Low urine output	IVP or ultrasound Occluded catheter	Placement of ureteral catheter or percutaneous nephrostomy
Urinary extravasation	Fever Abdominal pain or distension Low urine output	IVP, or ultrasound, or catheter injection	Ureteral catheter, percutaneous nephrostomy, or open drainage

Should the drainage from the catheter decrease, the initial step is to gently irrigate the ureteral catheter with 3 to 5 ml. of saline. Failure to remedy the problem by this method usually implies either displacement of the catheter or extravasation of urine proximal to the catheter tip. In these instances, the patient should be taken to the radiology department for contrast injection studies under fluoroscopy.

Patency of the catheters is essential, especially if the ureteral wall has been weakened or injured by stone manipulation or endoscopic resection. If the catheters are obstructed by blood, debris, or mechanical problems, an undue amount of pressure develops within the collecting system. This pressure could cause perforation, with massive urinary extravasation through the previously weakened ureteral wall.

An alternative to the use of standard ureteral catheters is the use of internal ureteral stents. We have found the routine use of small-caliber, self-retaining stents to be very satisfactory after the uncomplicated removal of an upper urinary tract calculus.

It appears that patients so treated have shorter hospital stays and that they have less discomfort. Elderly men, who may be expected to have a high intravesical voiding pressure, should have an intravesical catheter for 24 to 48 hours even with an indwelling stent in order to minimize reflux into the treated ureter. Flexible cystoscopy is then used to remove the stent at the time of the first outpatient visit 2 to 6 weeks after stone removal.

Alternatively, a non-absorbable suture may be attached to the tip of the stent and left hanging from the urethra for stent removal.

Long-Term Patient Follow Up

Each patient who has undergone a ureteroscopic procedure is seen again as an outpatient 2 to 6 weeks and again at 3 months after stone removal. This does not include those patients undergoing ureteroscopic surveillance of an upper urinary tract tumor who are followed at 3-month intervals as inpatients.

During each return visit as an outpatient, the patient undergoes a complete history and physical examination. A urinalysis is also done at each visit. Further diagnostic studies are performed only if the patient's history or physical examination suggests a problem.

An excretory urogram is done on every patient within 3 to 6 months of the original procedure. Of course, if symptoms of ureteral origin become evident earlier, this study is done more urgently than if the patient remains totally asymptomatic. These films, when compared with pre-ureteroscopy radiographs, will confirm the integrity of upper tract anatomy and renal function.

CHAPTER 10

Ureteropyeloscopy with Flexible Fiberoptic Instruments

DEMETRIUS H. BAGLEY

Flexible ureteropyeloscopy has gained value and acceptance as an endoscopic technique largely as a result of the advances achieved with rigid ureteropyeloscopy. Flexible techniques remain particularly valuable for evaluation and treatment of intraluminal lesions of the upper urinary tract in selected patients. Although the instruments for flexible ureteropyeloscopy were available for clinical use before rigid instruments, the widespread application of flexible ureteroscopic techniques has been limited because of the relatively uncommon indications for their use in diagnosis, the limited instruments for interventional procedures, and the fragility and expense of the endoscopes. The greatest limitation has been the lack of working capability. Significant progress in each of these areas promises a marked expansion in the application of flexible ureteropyeloscopy.

Development of Flexible Ureteropyeloscopy

In 1964, visualization of a calculus in the distal ureter was reported.[1] The stone was seen with a flexible fiberoptic instrument containing viewing and illuminating fiberoptic bundles. The instrument, a 9-F fiberscope developed by American Cystoscope Makers, Inc., was not deflectable and had no provision for irrigation. It was passed through a 26-F cystoscope just as a ureteral catheter is.

Takagi and co-workers[2] reported their experience with a 2-mm. flexible fiberoptic ureteropyeloscope, the Olympus Model KF. This instrument also contained viewing and illuminating bundles but had no channel for irrigation. A 2.5-cm. section at the distal tip of the instrument could be angulated, which facilitated passage through the ureter. The authors indicated that the major difficulty encountered was in passing the instrument into the ureteral orifice. The instrument was often angulated sharply during attempts to pass the orifice, and breakage of the fibers resulted.

Takayasu and Aso[3] increased the success rate for insertion of the instrument from 80 to 100 per cent by using a flexible introducer sheath or guidetube. A special cystoscope designed with an ocular lens system protruding at a 45-degree angle from the shaft was used to minimize angulation of the flexible instrument. A special deflecting bridge was also employed to limit angulation. By this technique the guidetube was first passed through the cystoscope and engaged by the deflecting bridge. A ureteral catheter was then passed through the guidetube into the ureteral orifice, and the guidetube was subsequently advanced over the catheter into the distal ureter.

133

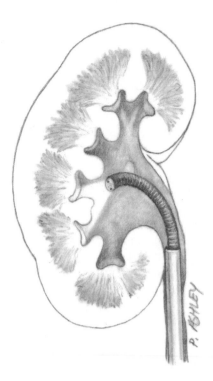

Figure 10–1. *The tip of the flexible ureteroscope has been passed through the sheath of a rigid ureteroscope, advanced into the pelvis, and angulated into the lower infundibulum.*

After removal of the ureteral catheter, the ureteropyeloscope was passed through the guidetube into the ureter. Thus, the ureteropyeloscope can be passed through this protective tube through the urethra and the bladder into the ureter itself. Irrigation could be provided only through the guidetube or by a diuresis to increase urinary flow. This type of irrigation offered some distension of the lumen, but it could clear only mild hematuria.

With the development of techniques for rigid ureteropyeloscopy, an ideal guidetube for entrance into the ureter became available. Bagley and co-workers[4] described the use of combined rigid and flexible ureteropyeloscopes. The rigid instrument could be used in the distal ureter and the more proximal portion into which it could pass. For inspection beyond a tortuosity that was particularly difficult to traverse or within the intrarenal collecting system, the flexible instrument (2.7 mm.) could be passed through the rigid sheath and used essentially as a flexible, deflectable telescope (Fig. 10–1). Irrigating fluid or working instruments could be passed through the outer rigid sheath.

The addition of an irrigating or working channel to the flexible ureteropyeloscope increases the size but sharply expands endoscopic visibility. Minimal bleeding no longer interferes with visibility if the blood can be cleared or diluted by irrigation. Deflection of the tip of the instrument provides maneuverability within the ureter and kidney thereby opening the calyces located laterally and inferiorly in the kidney to visual inspection during the same procedure.

The working capacity of the flexible ureteropyeloscopes remains minimal. The future development and expanded use of the flexible ureteropyeloscope depend upon the design of endoscopes that can be employed with working instruments that have the capability to obtain biopsy specimens, fragment and remove calculi, or destroy neoplastic tissue.

Instruments

Flexible ureteropyeloscopes possess, as their major distinguishing feature, flexibility. As with other endoscopes, they must possess a fiberoptic bundle for illumination and another for viewing. Flexibility, however, is the characteristic that allows the instrument to pass through a tortuous ureteral lumen or into the lateral intrarenal collecting system. Although this property is a major advantage, flexibility can also be a liability. The flexible ureteropyeloscope can generally be introduced easily through the cylindrical urethral lumen and may even be able to be passed into the ureteral orifice; however, it often buckles and coils within the larger lumen of the bladder as the tip encounters resistance in its passage within the ureter. Therefore, a major effort in development of these instruments has been directed toward maintaining flexibility, while affording them the rigidity needed for passage from the urethra to the ureter through the bladder.

TIP DESIGN

The design of the tip of the endoscope conveys many specific properties to the overall instrument. The tip may be of the same flexibility as the remainder of the shaft or it can be more or less flexible. It can also be molded into a specific configuration to allow passage into specific portions of the intrarenal collecting system. Directed deflectability of the tip conveys the greatest control and maneuverability but also significantly increases the size, the complexity, and the overall cost of the instrument.

PASSIVELY DEFLECTABLE FLEXIBLE ENDOSCOPES

A simple flexible endoscope without deflecting capability that is suitable for use as a ureteropyeloscope can be constructed at a relatively low cost. Several different manufacturers have designed such instruments, all with satisfactory illumination and visualization. The majority of these instruments have remained of little clinical value since they are not maneuverable and have no capacity for irrigation. Although the instrument can be placed directly into the ureter through an introducer sheath, the tip impinges directly on the mucosa and cannot be actively deflected into the lumen, and tortuous portions of the ureter often are not visualized. Irrigation can be provided through a secondary catheter if there is sufficient room for both instruments within the ureteral lumen.

Passively deflectable flexible endoscopes with a channel for irrigation provide better visualization because the irrigant is directed to clear the field of view. Instruments with an adequate channel may accept a guidewire, and thus can be directed along the ureteral lumen and afford better visibility. These instruments still have a limited range of motion within the renal pelvis and intrarenal collecting system.

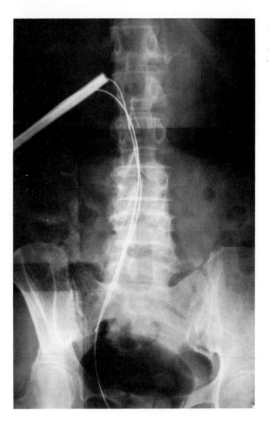

Figure 10–2. *This intraoperative abdominal radiograph demonstrates a rigid percutaneous nephroscope in place into the renal pelvis. A flexible ureteroscope is passed antegrade through the nephroscope into the ureter.*

Antegrade Ureteroscopy

A passively deflectable instrument can be introduced through an introducing catheter or sheath to the specific segment of ureter to be examined. We have employed this technique to examine the ureter after percutaneous removal of renal pelvic calculi (Fig. 10–2).[5] In this technique, a second guidewire is passed down the ureter in addition to the safety guidewire already in place. Over this secondary working guidewire is passed a standard 6-F ureteral dilator with an 8-F outer sheath or an 8-F dilator with a 10-F sheath. After the sheath has been passed into the proximal ureter, the inner dilator and the guidewire can be removed, leaving the empty sheath through which the flexible ureteroscope is passed.

Irrigation is necessary to distend the lumen and clear any debris from the field of view. We usually employ either a ureteral catheter that has been placed transurethrally into the ureteral orifice previously or an irrigating sheath (Fig. 10–3). The flexible instrument is then advanced along the ureter through this introducing sheath, and the ureter is inspected for any major fragments of calculus.

This technique has proved more useful in antegrade ureteroscopy than in retrograde ureteropyeloscopy. With the antegrade procedure, only the ureteral lumen is of interest and, the passively deflectable instrument provides satisfactory visualization within the limits of the ureteral lumen. However, in retrograde passage, the point of interest is often within the

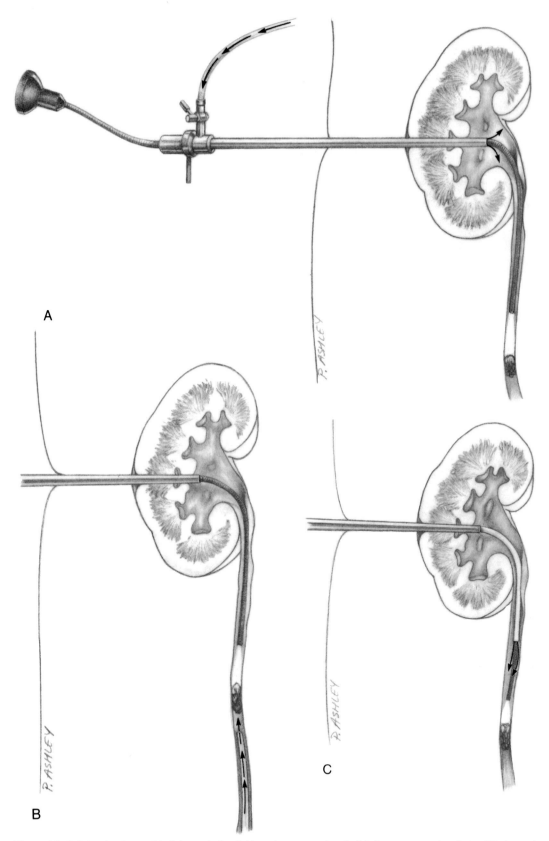

Figure 10–3. Irrigation is provided through the rigid nephroscope sheath (A), from a ureteral catheter (B), through the flexible irrigating sheath around the Flexiscope (C) or through a channel in the endoscope if that is available (D).

Illustration continued on following page

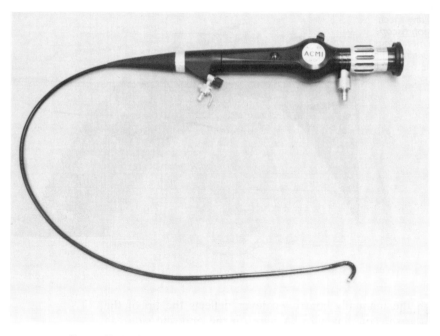

Figure 10–6. The ACMI flexible ureteropyeloscope.

Deflectability can also be obtained by placing a non-deflectable endoscope within a deflectable catheter. Catheters that can be steered have been available for radiologic applications for several years.* Deflectability is similarly conferred through a system of guidewires. A manually operated lever within the control unit pulls or releases opposing wires to deflect the tip of the instrument. This mechanism requires considerable space, and thus, the steerable catheter is several French sizes larger than the available lumen. The ureteropyeloscope therefore becomes a larger instrument that is more difficult to pass into the ureter; frequently it cannot be placed through the undilated ureter.

A third design utilizes an otherwise non-deflectable endoscope containing a 1-mm. channel in addition to the fiberoptic bundles for illumination and visualization. A deflectable guidewire similar to those used for years in deflectable brushes can be placed into the channel within the instrument to deflect the tip. Thus, as the instrument passes through the ureter or within the intrarenal collecting system, the tip can be deflected in one direction in any plane. The direction can be altered by turning the torque-controlled wire. This design has proved the least expensive and provides satisfactory deflectability in many circumstances.

"DISPOSABLE" ENDOSCOPES

Since flexible fiberoptic ureteropyeloscopes are extremely small and very fragile, one manufacturer has introduced the concept of disposable

---

*Medi-Tech, Watertown, MA.

instruments.* The flexible fiberoptic portion is designed separately from the ocular lens and control section (Fig. 10–7). The relatively inexpensive fiberoptic portions can then be replaced as they wear, while the more expensive but more durable ocular lens and control section can be used interchangeably with several different tips. A variety of flexible sections are available. Several of these instruments have two channels, one for irrigation, and a second for working instruments. Their role in flexible ureteropyeloscopy remains to be determined as these instruments become available to more practitioners.

Techniques for Passing the Flexible Ureteropyeloscope

One of the major difficulties encountered with flexible ureteropyeloscopes has been the need to obtain sufficient flexibility for full maneuverability and mobility within the ureter and the intrarenal collecting system while maintaining sufficient rigidity to provide for the instrument to be advanced manually through the urethra and the bladder into the ureter. Several techniques have been developed to facilitate passage through the bladder into the ureter.

---

*Van-Tec, Inc., P.O. Box 26, Spencer, IN 47460

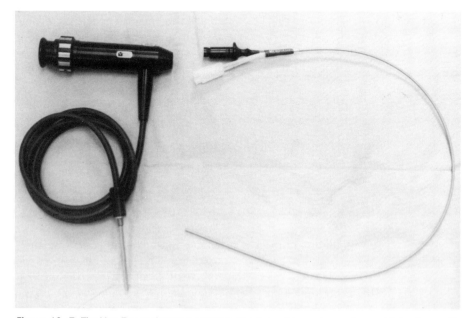

Figure 10–7. The Van-Tec endoscope consists of a focusable ocular portion and interchangeable objective tips of either rigid or flexible design.

DIRECT PASSAGE

The more rigid or stiffer flexible ureteropyeloscopes can occasionally be passed through the urethra and the bladder into a dilated ureter. A sufficiently rigid but still flexible instrument that encounters little resistance within the ureter may not buckle within the bladder as it passes from the urethra into the ureter. In a female, the instrument can be passed through the short urethra and directly toward the orifice with less risk of coiling than in the male urethra.

Few of the flexible ureteropyeloscopes available even as prototypes are sufficiently rigid to pass directly into the ureter in this way. Additional stiffness may be imparted to instruments that have a working channel by placing a stiff guidewire such as a Lunderquist wire into the working channel. This wire can remain within the channel and not be advanced directly into the ureter as it is with a standard guidewire technique (see later section).

CYSTOSCOPE AS GUIDETUBE

The sheath of the cystoscope used for dilating the ureteral orifice can be left within the bladder to serve as a rigid guidetube and to prevent coiling within the bladder. When the flexible instrument is to be passed into the ureter, the cystoscope is positioned at the ureteral orifice, and the telescope is removed (Fig. 10–8). The flexible instrument is then passed through the sheath of the cystoscope, preferably through a rubber gasket to seal the sheath as the ureteroscope is advanced through the sheath into the orifice. Therefore, the flexible instrument is contained within the cystoscope sheath and cannot coil within the larger lumen of the bladder. In order to maintain a usable conduit, the sheath of the cystoscope must be held near the ureteral orifice throughout the procedure. This is physically difficult and cumbersome and should be avoided if other more efficient techniques are available.

The more rugged flexible instruments can be passed through the working channel of the cystoscope and advanced into the orifice under direct visual control. It is usually much easier to place the endoscope in this way and more convenient to maintain the position of the cystoscope sheath (Fig. 10–9).

The short ureteroscope can also function as a rigid introducer sheath. After it has been placed into the distal ureter under direct vision, the telescope can be removed and the flexible instrument passed through the lumen. Thus, the rigid sheath provides a more stable conduit to the ureteral lumen (Fig. 10–10).

COMBINED RIGID AND FLEXIBLE URETEROPYELOSCOPY

Combining the small flexible ureteropyeloscope with the rigid ureteropyeloscope has been very successful. The flexible instrument can function as a flexible telescope within the rigid sheath. Thus, the endoscopic reach of the ureteropyeloscope is extended from the limits of the forward viewing or the lateral viewing telescope into otherwise inaccessible portions of the intrarenal collecting system.

Figure 10–8. The flexible ureteropyeloscope is passed through the sheath of the cystoscope into the orifice. Thus, the sheath of the cystoscope functions as a rigid guidetube.

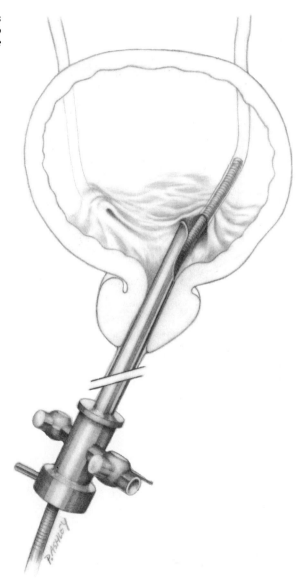

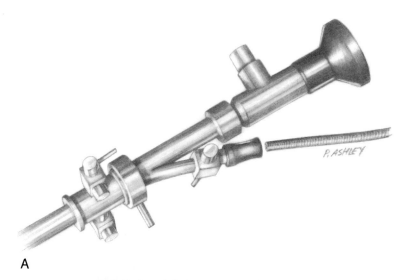

A

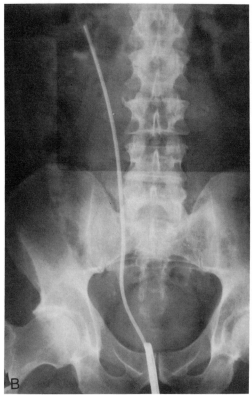

B

Figure 10–9. A, The Schott ureteroscope can be passed through the working channel of a 23 F cystoscope and placed under direct vision into the orifice. B, A radiograph of the abdomen shows the instrument after it has been passed to the level of the renal pelvis.

Figure 10–10. The short ureteroscope can be passed into the distal ureter, where it functions as a guidetube for introduction of the flexible ureteroscope.

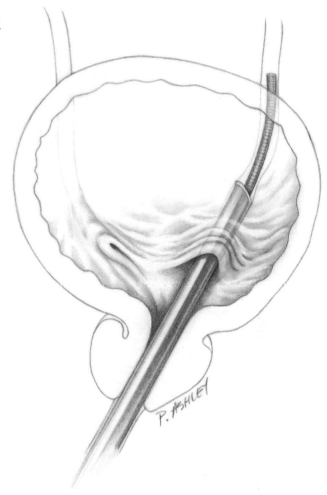

The combination can be used by first placing the rigid ureteropyeloscope into the ureter by the techniques discussed earlier (see Chapter 7). As the rigid instrument reaches its limits of passage because of a narrow or tortuous portion of the ureter or because of its location within the renal pelvis, the telescope can be removed and a small flexible ureteropyeloscope passed through the rubber gasket into the rigid sheath (Fig. 10–11). Thus, irrigation can be obtained through the sheath and the 5-F working channel remains available for secondary working instruments. As the flexible instrument is passed beyond the rigid sheath, the tip can be deflected to traverse a tortuous ureter or to view within the renal pelvis or to enter otherwise inaccessible infundibula (see Fig. 10–1).

This technique has been very successful in several patients.[4, 6] It combines the major advantages of each of the techniques of ureteropyeloscopy. The superior optics of the rigid instrument are used to inspect the accessible portion of the upper urinary tract while the rigid sheath is used to direct the flexible instrument through the bladder and into the ureter before its capability for flexibility and deflection are employed within the intrarenal collecting system.

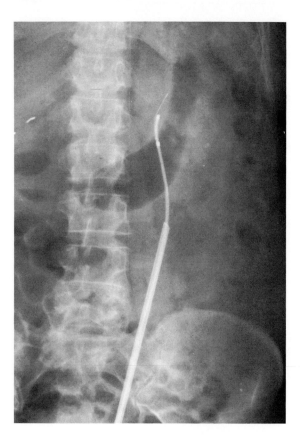

Figure 10–11. *The flexible ureteropyeloscope has been passed through the rigid ureteroscope sheath, and a deflectable brush has been placed through the working channel in the same rigid sheath. The brush can then be manipulated independently but placed under vision.*

Working instruments such as a deflectable brush, snare, or grasper can be used with the combination of the flexible and rigid ureteropyeloscopes (Fig. 10–11). A 5-F instrument can be passed through the working channel of the rigid sheath and placed with fluoroscopic guidance into the area to which the flexible endoscope is directed. As the working instrument comes into view through the flexible endoscope, both can be individually manipulated to perform the working tasks under vision. The independent manipulation of these two instruments affords a somewhat greater range of visual control. Since the working instrument is not limited to a single field of the endoscope, even greater visual control may result.

FLEXIBLE GUIDETUBE

A flexible guidetube can be employed to direct the ureteropyeloscope from the urethra into the ureter. A Teflon guidetube can be loaded onto a graduated ureteral dilator, which is advanced over a guidewire into the ureter (Fig. 10–12). The dilator and guidewire are then removed, leaving a lumen through the flexible guidetube into the ureter. The selected flexible endoscope is passed through the guidetube into the ureter. When an endoscope with a working or irrigation channel is used, irrigation can be passed directly through the flexible instrument and allowed to drain from the ureter along the guidetube. If no working channel is available within the

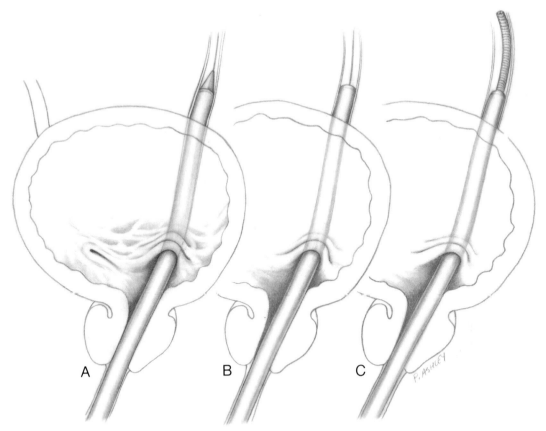

Figure 10–12. A, A flexible guidetube is passed over a graduated flexible ureteral dilator into the distal ureter. B. The guidewire may be left in place as the dilator is removed, or both the guidewire and dilator can be removed (C), leaving the sheath as a conduit from the urethra into the ureter for the flexible ureteroscope.

endoscope, then irrigation can be provided by passing a ureteral catheter alongside the endoscope within the guidetube or by using a semi-occlusive rubber gasket with a side arm at the outer portion of the guidetube.

Some difficulty may be encountered in advancing the guidetube within the ureter. This may be overcome by first dilating the ureter at least two French sizes larger than the external dimension of the guidetube. Since the guidetubes are relatively soft, some kinking may be encountered. If the wall of the guidetube is visualized as the flexible endoscope is advanced, the kink can be relieved by gently withdrawing the guidetube for a short distance. As the lumen opens, the endoscope is again advanced.

GUIDEWIRE

A guidewire can be used to direct certain flexible instruments into the ureteral orifice (Fig. 10–13). Only endoscopes that have a channel appropriate to accept a standard flexible guidewire can be used with this technique. After cystoscopic dilation of the ureterovesical junction, the guidewire is left in place within the ureter or, if desired, a second working guidewire can be placed into the ureter, so that the first guidewire acts as a safety wire. The

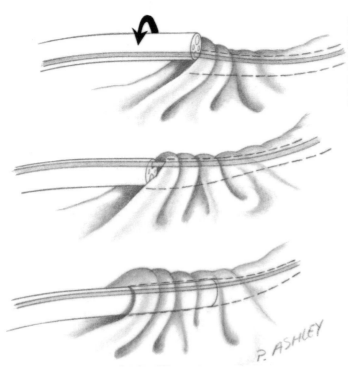

Figure 10–13. A guidewire can be used to guide flexible endoscopes into the ureteral orifice. Care should be taken as the tip approaches the orifice. Since the channel is located eccentrically at the tip of the instrument, it may impinge upon the lip of the orifice. The instrument should be turned to allow it to pass into the lumen.

cystoscope is then removed, leaving the ureteral guidewire protruding through the urethra. The flexible endoscope is placed over the guidewire by passing the guidewire in a retrograde fashion through the working channel of the instrument. The urologist advances the endoscope over the guidewire as an assistant holds the wire firmly.

The operator can see through the instrument as it passes through the urethra and the bladder into the ureteral orifice. It is very helpful to view the orifice through the endoscope as the ureteroscope is inserted so that the instrument can be oriented to fit best into the orifice. Since the working channel is usually eccentrically placed in the cross-section of the instrument, it is usually easier to place the larger portion of the tip posteriorly at the orifice to prevent it from impinging on the overhanging lip of the anterior wall of the intravesical ureter (Fig. 10–13). Within the ureter, the tip of the instrument will follow the guidewire and the course of the ureteral lumen. The wire must remain in place as the instrument is passed through the ureter, since the portion within the bladder may coil rather than enter the ureter. Coiling may occur even with a guidewire in place. Although we prefer to start with a standard 0.038-inch, heavy-duty, straight, floppy-tipped guidewire, it may be necessary to replace this with a much stiffer wire such as a Lunderquist wire. As the instrument reaches the renal pelvis, it may be possible to remove the guidewire and manipulate the instrument within the intrarenal collecting system with the channel free for irrigation or working instruments.

Passing the Ureteropyeloscope

THE URETER

After the flexible ureteropyeloscope has been placed into the distal ureter with one of the techniques described, it can usually be passed directly within the ureteral lumen. A guidetube or guidewire used for placing the ureteropyeloscope into the orifice must be maintained in the correct position as the instrument is passed through the ureter because the resistance between the instrument and the lumen is usually enough to cause the instrument to buckle and coil within the free lumen of the bladder if such movement is not actively prevented.

Other impediments to passage may also be encountered. Tortuosities within the ureter may be relatively difficult to pass. It is helpful to maintain the lumen within the field of view by manipulating the tip of the instrument appropriately. Irrigation into the ureter distends the lumen and may partially straighten a tortuosity. Radiographic contrast material added to the irrigant outlines the lumen for fluoroscopic visualization. The direction of curvature of the ureter is then obvious, and the appropriate direction for deflecting the tip is immediately anticipated. If the lumen of the ureter has been inspected previously, then the instrument can be passed through the ureter with radiologic monitoring alone. Thus, it is passed just as a ureteral catheter is placed, under fluoroscopic vision.

Narrow, non-distensible segments within the ureter may also be encountered. Although the flexible instruments are usually of a smaller caliber than the rigid ureteropyeloscopes, these regions may be sufficiently small to impede passage of the endoscope. This problem can usually be anticipated by performing a retrograde pyelogram to locate any non-distensible segments. Those areas can then be dilated with one of the techniques described in Chapter 5. Particular care should be taken during dilating these areas for flexible ureteropyeloscopy because of the limited irrigation capability of the flexible instruments. It may be very difficult to clear excessive blood from within the lumen for adequate visualization.

THE INTRARENAL COLLECTING SYSTEM

As the tip of the instrument enters the renal pelvis, the operator is confronted by numerous undefined ostia of infundibula within the visual field. The ureteropelvic junction is usually the only defined landmark. In the unusual case of a bifid pelvis, orientation is much easier; but it is usually extremely difficult to define or locate individual infundibula (Fig. 10–14).

Fluoroscopic monitoring is essential for this portion of the procedure. Radiographic contrast material (30%) should be introduced into the lumen so that the outline of the collecting system is visible radiographically. The instrument is located more easily radiographically than endoscopically. The radiographic location should be correlated with the endoscopic appearance so that landmarks within the collecting system can be recognized. A flexible guidewire within the lumen also provides a landmark that can be recognized

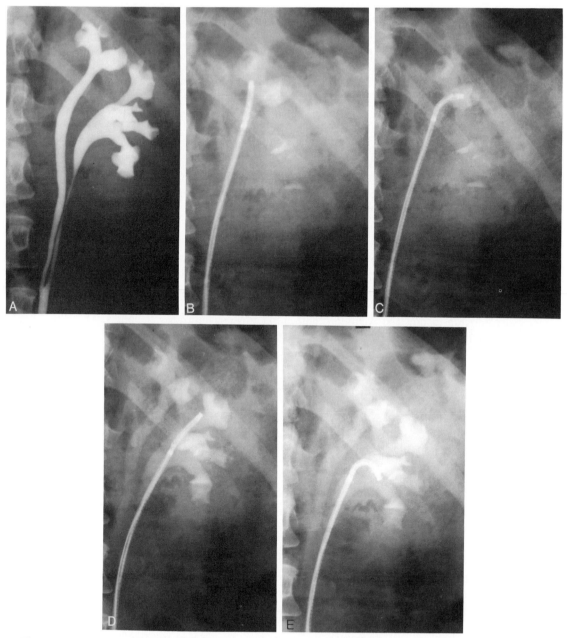

Figure 10–14. A retrograde ureteropyelogram demonstrates a duplicated intrarenal collecting system (A). Radiographs direct and confirm placement of a deflectable, flexible ureteroscope into different portions of the superior (B and C) and inferior (D and E) areas of the collecting system, which are opacified by irrigation with radiographic contrast material.

both fluoroscopically and endoscopically. As the ureteropyeloscope passes from the ureter, it usually courses into the infundibulum to the upper pole.

The particular technique used for inspecting the intrarenal collecting system varies with the purpose of the procedure. Evaluation of gross hematuria or abnormal cytologic study results demands thorough inspection of the urothelial surface. Inspection should be started within the pelvis as the instrument enters from the ureteropelvic junction. The infundibula should then be inspected sequentially. It is easier to start with a readily recognizable infundibulum, usually the upper pole infundibulum and calyces and then progress to the other more inferiorly located infundibula. Preoperative radiographs with contrast should be available to allow confirmation of the anatomy seen fluoroscopically.

If a specific lesion within the intrarenal collecting system is to be inspected or manipulated, then it should be sought directly. The lesion that has been located specifically on preoperative radiographs should be the same area located fluoroscopically at the time of the procedure. The best approach to visualize that area can then be determined. As noted, the upper pole is usually the easiest to reach with the flexible ureteropyeloscope. Conversely, the lower pole infundibula are the most difficult to enter. Although the ostia can usually be visualized with the instrument at the level of the pelvis and the instrument deflected toward the lower pole, it is more difficult to pass the ureteropyeloscope directly into the infundibula. It is often possible, particularly with an instrument with a secondary bending section, to pass excess length of the instrument into the renal pelvis, deflect the tip, and bounce it off the cephalad portion of the renal pelvis in order to press the tip into the lower pole infundibula. In our series of patients evaluated with deflectable, flexible ureteropyeloscopes, the entire intrarenal collecting system could be visualized in 83 per cent.[6]

WORKING WITHIN THE INTRARENAL COLLECTING SYSTEM

Very few working instruments and techniques are available for use within the intrarenal collecting system with the flexible ureteropyeloscopes. Deflectable instruments that will pass through the working channel of the rigid ureteropyeloscope can be used alongside the smaller flexible endoscopes. The working instrument and the endoscope must be deflected separately to pass into the area of interest. Again, fluoroscopic vision is essential. When placed within the field of view of the flexible ureteropyeloscope, the working instrument can be used under direct vision. Thus, the accuracy of brushing or grasping, or the removal of the proper biopsy specimen, can be monitored visually during the procedure. The deflectable working instruments can be used similarly through a flexible guidetube if it is of sufficient caliber to accept both the endoscope and the working instrument. Only the simplest instruments such as a brush or a snare are available to pass through a 3- or 3.5-F working channel of a flexible ureteropyeloscope. The larger instruments with a 4- or 5-F working channel can accommodate a wider range of more significant instruments (Fig. 10–15). Various graspers and baskets can be employed, but their uses are limited to the visual field afforded by the integral working channel of the instrument. Successful use of the flexible ureteropyeloscope for therapeutic

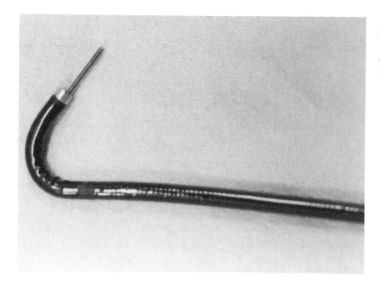

Figure 10–15. *A 3.5 F electrohy-draulic lithotriptor probe is positioned within the 4.2 F working channel of the ACMI flexible ureteropyeloscope.*

procedures awaits the development of more useful working instruments that will fit in the ureter alongside or within the flexible endoscopes.

At the completion of the procedure, the instrument is withdrawn through the lumen. Particular care should be taken to make certain that the tip of the instrument is straight as it is withdrawn into a guidetube or particularly into the rigid sheath. If the instrument is forcibly withdrawn as the tip is angulated, then the edge of the sheath may damage the flexible instrument.

Post-Operative Drainage

A ureteral catheter is inserted to the level of the renal pelvis after the procedure. We prefer an open-end ureteral catheter that can accept a guidewire if it is necessary to reposition the catheter later or exchange it for a self-retaining stent. The catheter can usually be passed easily through the guidetube or sheath of the ureteropyeloscope. Alternatively, if a safety guidewire has been left in place, the catheter can be passed over that guidewire or another catheter can be passed through the guidetube or sheath into the upper portion of the system. A 4.8-F, self-retaining diversionary catheter has also become available, which fits through the working channel of the rigid ureteropyeloscope and can be passed under direct vision. It will also pass through the working channel of the larger flexible instruments. The ureteral catheter must then be secured to a Foley catheter within the bladder to prevent its movement. The catheter is left in place from 24 to 72 hours or until any gross hematuria clears.

Irrigation

Irrigation is advantageous to distend the lumen of the ureter and the intrarenal collecting system and to dilute any blood within the lumen. In using different techniques for flexible ureteropyeloscopy, we have made every effort to provide for active irrigation. Intraluminal visualization has been distinctly superior during active irrigation.

Physiologic saline should be used as the irrigant for any ureteral or renal endoscopic procedure, since systemic absorption may occur via pyelolymphatic or pyelovenous backflow. The pressure for irrigation should be maintained at less than 30 cm. of water to minimize the chance of absorption.

Some authors working with only the small flexible endoscopes have not used irrigation but rather relied upon fluid diuresis to provide a physiologic irrigant and luminal distension.

Peri-Operative Care

Appropriate peri-operative care of patients for flexible ureteropyeloscopy must include careful selection of appropriate patients. Since this is a new procedure, the urologist's diagnostic or therapeutic goal must be carefully defined, with the limitations of the instruments in mind. Patients should be fully informed of the procedure and its objectives. Alternative diagnostic techniques such as open surgical exploration or watchful waiting before repeating other more conventional procedures should also be explained to the patient.

Anesthesia has been essential for flexible ureteropyeloscopy by the techniques described because the ureterovesical junction is dilated, causing pain, and because distension of the intrarenal collecting system may occur with irrigation. We have preferred general anesthesia since it provides good relaxation with total anesthesia and also provides for controlled respiration so that movement of the kidney can be managed by the anesthesiologist. Spinal anesthesia is also satisfactory but provides only a limited time for performing the procedure and also does not allow respiratory control. Epidural techniques provide a more variable period of anesthesia but also do not control respiration. We have used the smaller flexible instruments without ureteral dilation and with manual irrigation in some patients under local anesthesia.

Systemic antibiotics have been given on a prophylactic basis in the perioperative period. Although no controlled studies have been undertaken or demonstrated a benefit of such therapy, the risk of contamination and the potential for pyelovenous and pyelolymphatic backflow supports such administration.

Post-operatively, a ureteral catheter is left in place to drain the upper urinary tract for 24 to 72 hours. This catheter provides for drainage past an edematous segment of the ureter and past intraluminal clots. It is generally left in place until the urinary drainage is clear. Analgesics are available as necessary should the patient develop any discomfort following removal of the catheter. Alternatively, a self-retaining ureteral stent (e.g., a double pigtail catheter) could be placed to allow earlier discharge of the patient. Standard monitoring of the patient's vital signs and clinical course should be initiated immediately after endoscopy and maintained while the ureteral catheter is in place.

Table 10–1
PATIENTS EVALUATED WITH FLEXIBLE URETEROPYELOSCOPY*

Indications	No. of Patients	Endoscope Passed to Kidney (No. of Patients)	No. of Successful Procedures
Filling Defect ± Hematuria	23	23	23
Hematuria	21	17	9
? Tumor	6	5	5
? Calculus	4	4	4
Obstructed UPJ†	3	3	3
TOTAL	57	52	44

*Reprinted with permission from Bagley DH, Huffman JL, and Lyon ES: Flexible ureteropyelos-copy: Diagnosis and treatment in the upper urinary tract. J Urol. (In press).
  †UPJ = ureteropelvic junction.

Results of Flexible Ureteropyeloscopy

Flexible ureteropyeloscopy has proved to be of value in certain groups of patients. Patients with an upper urinary tract filling defect with or without hematuria were successfully instrumented with deflectable, flexible endo-scopes, and a diagnosis was achieved in 100 per cent (23 of 23) of cases (Table 10–1).[6] In each instance the presence or absence of a filling defect and the nature of that lesion could be determined. Less success was achieved with flexible instrumentation for evaluation of unilateral gross hematuria. A diagnosis was achieved in approximatley 50 per cent (9 of 17) of these patients. Other authors have had similar or lower success rates.[7, 8] The failures may have resulted from an inability to inspect the entire intrarenal collecting system, from an intraparenchymal source of bleeding, or from failure to recognize surface lesions responsible for the hematuria.

The non-deflectable, flexible ureteroscopes have also been of value in selected patients. The lumen of the ureter, the medial portion of the renal pelvis, and, in some patients, the upper infundibulum can be visualized. When the point of interest is in those areas, one of these simpler, less expensive endoscopic techniques will often suffice. The lateral portion of the intrarenal collecting system in most kidneys and the lower pole in essentially all kidneys is accessible only with a fully deflectable instrument.[8, 9, 10]

Others[11] have reported the value of percutaneous flexible nephroscopy in evaluation of patients with gross hematuria. Patterson and co-workers described "red spots" on the urothelium that could be fulgurated; fulguration then resulted in cessation of hematuria. Similar red spots may be induced by the trauma of instrumentation, including placement of the flexible guidewire, and may have been overlooked in our series.[6] Since Jardin[7] has not dilated the ureteral orifice in his patients, it is less likely a factor in his series.

Flexible ureteropyeloscopy has also been useful in searching for recur-rent upper urothelial tumors or intrarenal calculi. Larger series are necessary to determine the true value in these patients.

Application of Flexible Ureteropyeloscopy

Flexible ureteropyeloscopy should be employed in certain carefully selected patients. It provides many technical advantages not achieved with other endoscopic techniques or with more conventional radiologic techniques. It provides special advantages for evaluation of filling defects of the upper urinary tract. The development of small instruments that can be passed as easily as an ureteral catheter may render endoscopy the technique of first choice in evaluation of filling defects. Because it combines endoscopic visualization with maneuverability, flexible ureteropyeloscopy is ideal for bypassing ureteral configurations inaccessible to the rigid instruments and for endoscopic access to the intrarenal collecting system.

References

1. Marshall VF: Fiberoptics in urology. J Urol 91:110, 1964.
2. Takagi T, Go T, Takayasu H, and Aso Y: Fiberoptic pyeloureteroscope. Surgery 70:661, 1971.
3. Takayasu H and Aso Y: Recent development for pyeloureteroscopy: guide tube method for its introduction into the ureter. J Urol 112:176, 1974.
4. Bagley DH, Huffman JL, and Lyon ES: Combined rigid and flexible ureteropyeloscopy. J Urol 130:243, 1983.
5. Bagley DH and Rittenberg MH: Percutaneous antegrade flexible ureteroscopy. Urology 27:331, 1986.
6. Bagley DH, Huffman JL, and Lyon ES: Flexible ureteropyeloscopy: Diagnosis and treatment in the upper urinary tract. J Urol (in press).
7. Jardin A: Flexible trans-urethral ureterorenoscopy. Presented at the Third Congress of the International Society of Urologic Endoscopy. Karlsruhe, Federal Republic of Germany, August 1984.
8. Aso Y, Ohtawara YI, Suzuki K, Tajima A, and Fujita K: Usefulness of fiberoptic pyeloureteroscope in the diagnosis of the upper urinary tract lesions. Urol Int 39:355, 1984.
9. Bagley DH: Ureteral endoscopy with passively deflectable, irrigating flexible ureteroscopes. Urology 29:170, 1987.
10. Bagley DH: Flexible ureteropyeloscopy with modular, "disposable" endoscope. Urology 29:296, 1987.
11. Patterson D, Segura JW, Benson RC Jr, Leroy AJ, and Wagoner R: Endoscopic evaluation and treatment of patients with idiopathic gross hematuria. J Urol 132:1199, 1984.

CHAPTER 11

Complications of Ureteropyeloscopy

R. ERNEST SOSA
DEMETRIUS H. BAGLEY
JEFFRY L. HUFFMAN

Ureteropyeloscopy is a potentially hazardous procedure. The delicate, thin-walled ureter is vulnerable to trauma at all stages of endoscopic intervention, from the dilation of the intramural ureter to the final removal of the ureteroscope. Most complications (Table 11–1) result from mechanical injury to the ureter during manipulation, but significant morbidity may result from endoscopy in a patient with infected urine, or from the introduction of infection at the time of endoscopy. The extravasation of irrigation fluid may also lead to serious morbidity. In the hands of the experienced groups reporting at the Third Congress of the International Society of Urologic Endoscopy in Karlsruhe, 1984, there were 38 complications in 838 uretero-pyeloscopic procedures, for a complication rate of 4.5 per cent (Table 11–2).[1] No deaths or loss of renal units were reported.

Early Complications

PERFORATION

Mechanical injury of the ureter at the time of the ureteroscopic proce-dure comprised 71 per cent of the reported complications. Most of these injuries are resolved by the placement of an indwelling ureteral catheter for an appropriate period of time. Less than 10 per cent of the patients in this report suffered complications requiring surgical correction of their injuries.

The most frequent injury was the disruption of the ureteral mucosa without evident perforation on visual inspection. However, in many of these cases, contrast material can be shown to extravasate by intra-operative retrograde pyelography (Fig. 11–1 and 11–2). This injury will usually resolve by placing a stent in the ureter for 4 to 6 weeks.

A small perforation of the ureter evident on visual inspection may also be treated in this manner, reserving surgical correction for the larger ureteral disruptions and avulsions and for lesser injuries that do not respond to more conservative treatment.

Ureteral stents should be used following all ureteroscopic procedures in which manipulation of the ureter for removal of a stone or dilation of a stricture has taken place. The length of time that a stent should remain indwelling depends on the degree of trauma suffered by the ureter. As a guideline, we leave an indwelling ureteral catheter in place for 24 to 48 hours following a routine procedure for ureteral stone removal. The stent guards the patient against ureteral obstruction due to mucosal edema and/or

Table 11–1
POSSIBLE COMPLICATIONS OF URETEROPYELOSCOPY

Ureteral Injury
  Bleeding
  Thermal Injury
  Stricture
  Vesicoureteral Reflux
  Mucosal Tear
  False Passage
  Ureteral Perforation
  Ureteral Avulsion
  Periureteral Fluid Collection
    1. Hematoma
      a. Sterile
      b. Infected
    2. Extravasation of Irrigation Fluid
      a. Fluid Overload
      b. Dilutional Hyponatremia
      c. Hypo-Osmolarity with Hemolysis
      d. Infected Fluid Collection
Infection
  Urethritis
  Prostatitis
  Cystitis
  Pyelonephritis
  Bacteremia
  Sepsis
Instrument Breakage

Table 11–2
COMPLICATIONS OF URETEROPYELOSCOPY*

Complication	No. of Cases	Percentage of All Complications
Mucosal Injury	13	34.2
Ureteral Perforation	7	18.4
Ureteral Bleeding	4	10.5
Extravasation	2	5.3
Stricture Formation	1	2.6
Infection	11	29.0
TOTALS		
No. of Cases	838	
Complications (%)	38 (4.5)	
Mechanical injury (%)	27 (71.0)	
Infection (%)	11 (29.0)	

*Compiled from the Third Congress of the International Society of Urologic Endoscopy, Karlsruhe, Federal Republic of Germany, August, 1984.

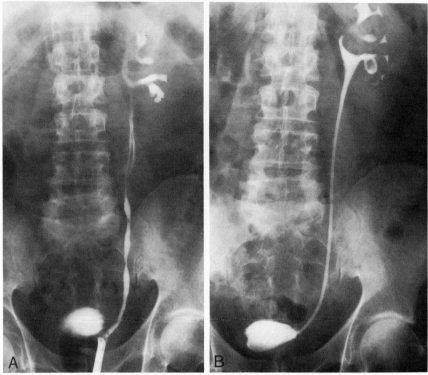

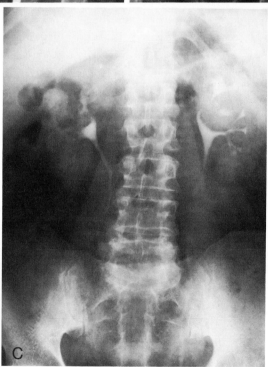

Figure 11–1. A, A patient with a persistent proximal ureteral calculus underwent uretero-pyeloscopic extraction of the stone after partial ultrasonic disintegration. There was a tight ureteral narrowing immediately distal to the calculus that required balloon dilation. A retrograde ureterogram done after the procedure revealed extravasation of contrast near the site of balloon dilation. B, A double pigtail ureteral stent was used post-operatively. This radiograph confirmed proper position of the stent in the left collecting system. C, Four weeks after the procedure, an excretory urogram was done. This revealed a normally functioning left kidney without evidence of extravasation or recurrent stricture formation at the site of the previous perforation.

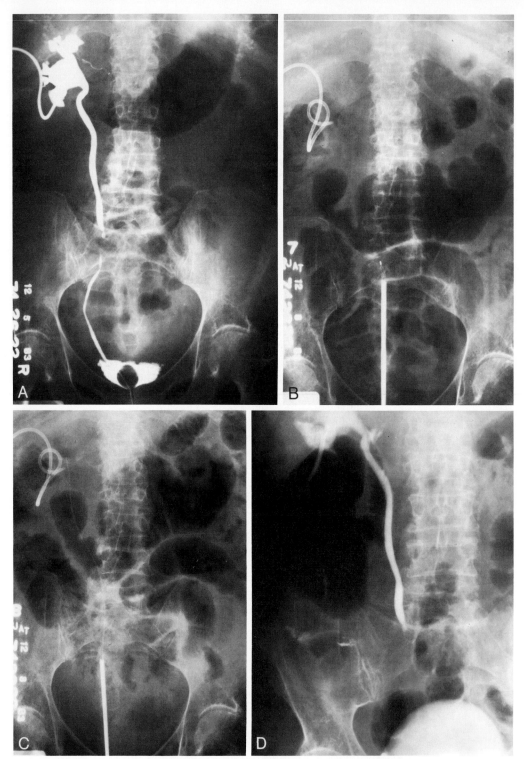

Figure 11–2. A, A 55-year-old woman presented with urinary tract sepsis and right hydronephrosis. A percutaneous nephrostomy tube was inserted. Several days later, an antegrade contrast study showed a partially obstructing mid-ureteral calculus with evidence of ureteral narrowing distal to the stone. B, The narrow segment in the ureter was dilated ureteropyeloscopically using a balloon catheter, and the stone was extracted intact. This radiograph shows the ureteropyeloscope in the mid ureter with a stone basket around the calculus. C, Mucosal disruption was noted near the site of balloon dilation, and a ureteral catheter was inserted using ureteropyeloscopic guidance. D, After removal of the ureteral catheter, an antegrade contrast study showed persistent blockage at the site of prior balloon dilation.

Illustration continued on opposite page

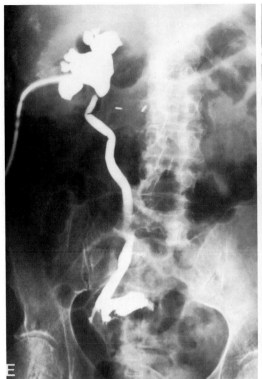

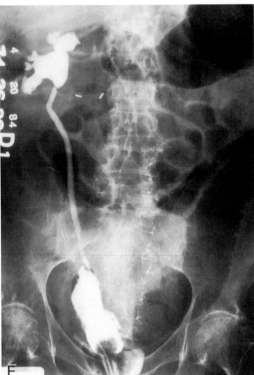

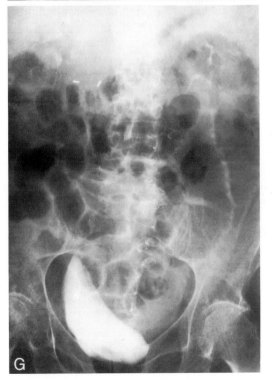

Figure 11–2 Continued E, *The nephrostomy tube was left in place, and the antegrade study was repeated in one month. This revealed extravasation of contrast from the previously obstructed site. F, A ureteral reimplant was performed using a psoas bladder hitch. After surgery, a cystogram demonstrated free reflux of contrast into the bladder, ureter, and kidney. G, A follow-up excretory urogram showed a normally functioning kidney without radiographic evidence of extravasation or obstruction.*

retained stone fragments. Balloon dilation of a tight and fibrotic ureteral stricture is traumatic, as the two case studies illustrate (see later section). Following dilation of a stricture, an indwelling catheter should remain in the ureter for 4 to 6 weeks to allow adequate time for healing.[2]

THERMAL INJURY

Avulsion of the ureter may also occur if one attempts to extract an oversized calculus without prior fragmentation. Ultrasonic lithotripsy has enhanced the efficacy and safety with which the ureteroscope can remove these larger calculi. More recently, the development of the offset viewing telescope permits application of the ultrasonic probe under direct vision, allowing the more purposeful destruction of a calculus. The main hazard in performing ultrasonic lithotripsy is thermal injury to the ureter by an overheated probe.[3] This complication is avoided by use of continuous flow irrigation during the procedure to keep the probe from overheating. Frequent monitoring of the probe's temperature by touch, taking rest periods to allow the probe to cool when necessary, is also important. Using the offset lens ureteroscope may make these precautions more difficult to follow. This probe has a smaller diameter than the probe utilized with the standard ureteroscope. The smaller size diminishes the efficacy of excess heat removal by continuous irrigation and increases the possibility that the probe's lumen will become blocked by stone particles or debris. Better irrigant flow can be established if the probe is used as the inflow port of irrigant and the ureteroscope sheath as the outflow port. In either case, care must be taken to ensure that continuous flow is maintained during ultrasonic lithotripsy. The offset lens eliminates the need to interchange the telescope and probe during lithotripsy. The endoscopist must remember to interrupt his or her progress periodically to check the probe's temperature. With either instrument, gentle execution of the lithotripsy will prevent unnecessary trauma to the ureter. Similarly, irrigation should be maintained during electrohydraulic lithotripsy in the ureter to avoid heat buildup.

EXTRAVASATION

The irrigant used for ureteroscopy may extravasate during the course of the procedure if significant trauma to the ureter occurs. The resultant morbidity is determined by the amount of fluid extravasated, the patient's general health, and the nature of the irrigation fluid. Fluid in the retroperitoneal space is readily absorbed into the vascular space. The absorption of a large volume of fluid can significantly alter plasma volume and composition. The absorption of normal saline will not produce changes in osmolarity or electrolyte composition, but could cause fluid overload. Glycine hyperabsorption does not produce changes in osmolarity but does produce a dilutional hyponatremia. Water is potentially the most dangerous irrigant, as its absorption can produce hemolysis, resulting in possible renal failure and death. Accordingly, the preferred irrigation fluid for ureteroscopy is normal saline unless electrocautery is to be used, in which case glycine is the irrigation fluid used.

A retroperitoneal collection of fluid can also be due to leakage of urine through a ureteral perforation, or it can represent a hematoma due to ureteral injury. In the former case, urine diversion by an indwelling ureteral catheter or percutaneous nephrostomy plus a ureteral stent left in place for 4 to 6 weeks will usually correct the problem. In the latter case, frequent assessment of the patient and hematocrit checks will help determine if conservative treatment or open intervention is indicated. In either case, a ureteral stent is necessary to assure that the urine is diverted from the site of injury and that the ureter remains patent.

INSTRUMENT BREAKAGE

The ureteropyeloscope sheath is designed to be atraumatic during its insertion into the small lumen of the ureter, while maintaining sufficient firmness to withstand the forces placed on it by the prostate gland, the psoas muscle, and the natural curvatures of the ureter itself. In some instruments the distal half of the sheath is smaller in size (~11.5 F) than the proximal portion (13 F), which must be firmer. At the juncture of these two segments there is a step-off that is subjected to stress as the ureteroscope is maneuvered. It is not unusual to note a curvature in the ureteroscope, most marked at this point, after use of the instrument in a few patients. It is precisely at this juncture that a ureteropyeloscope is most likely to break if one attempts to manually straighten the sheath (Fig. 11–3). A bent ureteroscope should

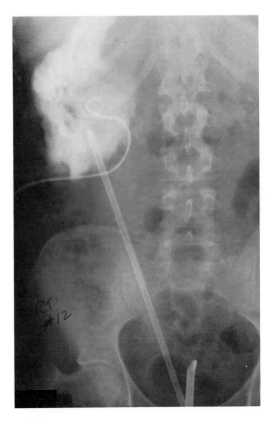

Figure 11–3. This radiograph shows a fractured ureteropyeloscope. The distal segment remains from the bladder into the ureter. A cystoscope is in the bladder. A percutaneous nephrostomy tube has been placed; however, a large amount of extravasation of contrast exists.

be returned to the manufacturer who can assess the soundness of the sheath and correct the defect. Another precaution that may be taken during ureteroscopy to avoid intraoperative fracture of the ureteroscope is to take notice of the circular field of vision through the telescope at the start of the procedure. If the circular shape becomes an oval shape as the instrument courses over the prostate or over the psoas muscle, then undue force is being placed on the sheath. Further insistence may result in fracture of the instrument. Accordingly, the procedure should be terminated and an alternative plan put into effect.

INFECTION

Symptomatic urinary tract or systemic infection afflicted 11 of 838 patients (1.3%) following ureteropyeloscopy. Bacteria present in the urinary tract are introduced into the renal parenchyma in a retrograde fashion by the pressure of the irrigation fluid. Systemic seeding by pyelolymphatic and pyelovenous backflow can then occur. To minimize the risk of endoscopy-associated infections, all patients should have negative pre-operative urine cultures as discussed in Chapter 4. The use of peri-operative prophylactic antibiotics even if negative urine culture results are obtained is recommended.

BLEEDING

The safe handling of the ureteroscope depends on the maintenance of good visibility at all times. If visibility is impaired owing to debris or to the introduction of air bubbles or to ureteral bleeding and cannot be regained by irrigation, endoscopy should be terminated immediately. Fortunately, obscured visibility due to debris, though a frequent occurrence, is readily corrected by gentle suction or irrigation with a small syringe attached to the side port of the instrument's sheath. Significant ureteral bleeding during ureteroscopy has been a rare occurrence; in fact, it was reported in only four patients of the 838 cases (less than 0.5%).

Late Complications

Limited data are available on long-term complications of ureteral pyeloscopy. Lyon and colleagues have reported on over 240 ureteroscopic procedures performed over 8 years with both flexible and rigid ureteropyeloscopes.[4, 5] They have not found any late upper urinary tract abnormalities due to ureteropyeloscopy even in patients undergoing multiple endoscopies. Twelve to 36 months after the ureteropyeloscopic procedures, Stackl and Marberger[6] performed urinalyses, cystograms, and excretory urograms in over 40 patients who had undergone ureteroscopic extraction of ureteral calculi from all locations in the ureter. They found no significant morphologic alterations of the upper urinary tracts such as ureteral stricture formation or loss of renal function in any patient.

However, in more recent reports, Lyon noted that three patients of over 240 developed ureteral strictures at the site of stone impaction after unusually long ultrasonic lithotripsy.[7] Biester and Gillenwater have commented on four patients with strictures after ureteroscopy and other procedures, two had long, narrow strictures of the upper ureter, one had a mid ureteral structure and one had a lower ureteral stricture.[8]

These preliminary reports indicate that most, if not all, complications will be detected in the early post-procedure period. However, careful follow up in all patients undergoing ureteroscopy is still strongly recommended.

Complications and the Learning Curve

The reported complication rate of 4.5 per cent is probably lower than the actual complication rate for all urologists performing ureteropyeloscopy. Endoscopists, during their early experience with ureteroscopy, may not report results. It is with initial procedures that authors of larger series have most complications. The reasons for the early difficulties are multifold. First, experience with endoscopy of the urethra and bladder is not sufficient by itself to endow proficiency in the use of the ureteropyeloscope. The ureter's small size and delicate nature render ureteropyeloscopy a more demanding procedure than cystoscopy, requiring compulsive adherence to the basic techniques described in prior chapters. Second, many urologists begin to perform ureteropyeloscopy before acquiring all the ancillary equipment necessary to use this instrument in an efficient and safe manner. Use of guidewires to introduce instruments into the ureter, ultrasonic lithotripsy to reduce stones to a less traumatizing size, and fluoroscopy for guidance during the execution of these procedures is imperative. However, with added experience, careful patient selection, adequate equipment, and proper execution of the basic techniques, complication rates will decline while success rates increase.

Examples of Ureteroscopic Complications

Patient No. 1. A 50-year-old male with a mid-ureteral stricture and a proximal calculus underwent ureteropyeloscopy. The stricture was dilated with a balloon catheter under fluoroscopic control, and the stone was fragmented by ultrasonic lithotripsy. Visual inspection of the ureter after removal of the stone revealed a small mucosal disruption at the site that had been dilated. An intra-operative retrograde pyelogram revealed the extravasation of contrast (see Fig. 11–1A). An indwelling double pigtail catheter was left in place for 4 weeks (see Fig. 11–1B). A follow-up excretory pyelogram (see Fig. 11–1C) reveals adequate healing of the injury.

Patient No. 2. A 55-year-old female known to have a small, right renal stone presented with complaints of right flank pain with fever, confused mental status, and hypotension. The patient had a long history of polymyositis and was receiving prednisone, 60 mg. daily, at the time of admission. After collection of blood and urine samples for culture and sensitivity, broad spectrum antibiotics were begun. Drainage of the obstructed kidney was established by prompt placement of a 12-F percutaneous nephrostomy tube. A transnephrostomy tube study, performed after the urine cultures were documented to show no growth, revealed a mid-ureteral stone proximal to a ureteral stricture (see Fig. 11–2A). The patient underwent ureteroscopy for stone extraction. The ureteral stricture was dilated with a balloon catheter, and the stone was removed by use of a basket (see Fig. 11–2B). Visual inspection of the ureter revealed a mucosal tear in the area of the stricture. Accordingly, a ureteral catheter was placed, and the nephrostomy tube was opened to gravity drainage (see Fig. 11–2C). Prednisone and antibiotics were continued post-operatively. The ureteral catheter was removed after 1 week. An antegrade pyelogram revealed an area of obstruction that was believed to represent mucosal edema (see Fig. 11–2D). The nephrostomy tube was kept open to drainage. Follow-up studies showed extravasation of a large amount of contrast material (see Fig. 11–2E). The patient was explored and underwent ureteral re-implantation into a psoas hitch (see Fig. 11–2F). At surgery, the friable nature of the patient's tissues secondary to long-term, high-dose steroid therapy was noted. An excretory pyelogram performed 2 months after the re-implantation revealed prompt bilateral renal function without hydronephrosis (see Fig. 11–2G). In this patient, an intra-operative retrograde pyelogram may have documented the presence of a small ureteral perforation. A ureteral catheter could have been left indwelling for 6 to 8 weeks initially, improving the likelihood of healing the injury without operative intervention.

References

1. The Third Congress of the International Society of Urologic Endoscopy, Karlsruhe, Federal Republic of Germany, August, 1984.
2. Banner MP, Pollack HM, Ring EJ, and Wein AJ: Catheter dilatation of benign strictures. Radiology 147:427, 1983.
3. Howards SS, et al: Ultrasonic lithotripsy. Invest Urol 11:272, 1974.
4. Lyon ES, Huffman JL, and Bagley DH: Ureteroscopy and ureteropyeloscopy. Urology 23:29, 1984.
5. Huffman JL, Bagley DH, and Lyon ES: Extending cystoscopic techniques into the ureter and renal pelvis—experience with ureteroscopy and pyeloscopy. JAMA 250:2002, 1983.
6. Stackl W and Marberger M: Late complications of the management of ureteral calculi with the ureterorenoscope. J Urol 136:386, 1986.
7. Lyon ES: Complications of ureteroscopy. Presented at the Third World Congress on Endourology, September 21, 1985.
8. Biester R and Gillenwater JY: Complications following ureteroscopy. J Urol 136:380, 1986.

CHAPTER 12

Care and Sterilization of Ureteropyeloscopic Instruments

DEMETRIUS H. BAGLEY

Ureteropyeloscopes are among the most fragile of urologic endoscopic instruments. The great length and small diameter of these instruments render them particularly vulnerable to damage. Each individual component of the instrument is similarly long and narrow and thus susceptible to breakage or malfunction. As an example, the working channel of the rigid, sheathed ureteropyeloscope is at most 5 F (<2 mm.); therefore, any particle, even those less than 1 mm. in diameter, within the lumen can cause significant obstruction.

The flexible ureteropyeloscopes are even more fragile. The very nature of their design and flexibility renders these instruments susceptible to angulation and kinking with resultant breakage. Since each fiber bundle is extremely small, it contains many fewer glass fibers than a larger instrument such as a nephroscope or a bronchoscope; therefore, loss of even a few fibers is much more noticeable and presents a greater visual loss in these instruments.

The ancillary working instruments also suffer from the fragility imposed by the demands of miniaturization. The stone baskets used with operating ureteropyeloscopes measure only 3.5 F, yet this retrieval device must include a sheath rigid enough to contain and close the three or four wires that form the basket. Each component of the instrument has been manufactured to minimal tolerances and demands the greatest care for continued function.

As with all endoscopic instruments, ureteropyeloscopes carry the risk of infection and cross contamination as they are introduced into the patients' body cavities. This risk is emphasized further since these instruments pass directly into the upper urinary system, traversing the defenses of the bladder and the ureterovesical junction.

Mechanical Cleaning

Mechanical cleaning of endoscopes after use is the most important step in both the care and the sterilization of these instruments. Particulate matter such as blood or fragments of tissue clinging to the instrument provides a nidus for infection by retaining high concentrations of bacteria and it also forms a site for corrosion of the instrument. Special care must be taken with ureteropyeloscopes since the instruments are small, and the main lumen, and particularly the working channel, is minute.

The external surfaces of the instrument should be washed in warm water containing a detergent. Any irregularities in the instruments such as the junction of the stopcock to the sheath should be cleaned with a soft cloth or a soft brush to remove all particles. The lumen must be cleaned with a flow of water and preferably with a small, soft, flexible brush. The lumens of the irrigation channels and working channels should be cleaned similarly with a flow of warm water.

Instruments that cannot be submerged for cleaning should be wiped on all surfaces with a wet cloth. The lumen of the working or irrigation channel should also be irrigated for cleansing and to provide unobstructed flow. Particular care should be taken to avoid getting water into any portion of the instrument that is not sealed against submersion. Even small amounts of water leaking into the unsealed optical portions of a flexible ureteropyeloscope, for instance, will result in severe damage to the instrument, rendering it unusable.

After the instrument has been cleansed with a detergent solution, it should be thoroughly rinsed with clean running water, then with distilled water. The instrument should be thoroughly dried with a clean, soft, dry cloth or in a jet of dry compressed gas. Abrasive cleansers and cleaning instruments should be avoided since they can roughen the surfaces of the endoscope. A detergent, usually a moderately low alkaline, low sudsing agent, should be employed in the cleaning process. The choice of a specific agent should be guided by the recommendations of the instrument manufacturer. Ordinary soap should be avoided, since it can form insoluble alkaline films that can coat the instrument.

The exposed lenses of telescopes can be cleaned with a cotton swab moistened with alcohol to remove adherent debris and any precipitate that may have formed on the surface of the lens from the irrigating solutions. Cleansing of the lens can be monitored by visual inspection through the instrument. No metal or abrasive agent should be used for cleaning the lenses because of the possibility of scratching their surfaces.

Ultrasonic Cleaning

Although standard operative surgical instruments can be cleaned routinely in an ultrasonic cleaning machine, such machines should be avoided for these delicate endoscopes. Ureteropyeloscopes can be cleaned more safely and just as thoroughly by hand. The ultrasonic units may be effective in cleaning the small working instruments such as biopsy forceps or graspers, since they can effectively remove particulate matter within the tiny irregularities of these instruments.

Storage of Ureteropyeloscopes

Processing of ureteropyeloscopes should include careful storage in a protective container to support the instrument and isolate it from damage during handling, sterilization, and storage.

After cleaning, the disassembled endoscope should be placed into foam-lined metal boxes of sufficient dimensions to provide for a lining of foam

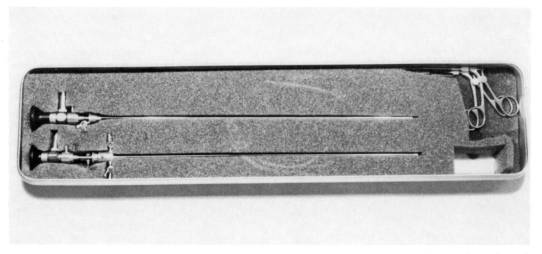

Figure 12–1. *The telescope and sheath are completely padded by form-fitting foam within a perforated metal case.*

between the instrument and the box on all sides. An effective design for padding is a sheet of foam into which slits have been cut to accept instruments of varying sizes (Fig. 12–1). The instruments should be disassembled, and the sheath and telescope should be placed separately within the padding. One manufacturer provides perforated metal tubing into which the telescopes can be fitted, thus offering an effective barrier to angulation or crushing of the long telescope (Fig. 12–2).

The flexible ureteropyeloscopes are even more difficult to protect adequately. They can be placed into a large, flat container of sufficient depth in a bed of foam padding. An egg carton designed pad is most effective for holding and separating the flexible portion of the instrument (Fig. 12–3). The ureteropyeloscope can be gently coiled within the container and held in this position to prevent movement of the tip during processing. Considerable care must be taken in handling these instruments, since the tip may fall from the container and will be damaged by any forceful angulation over the edge of the container.

Working instruments employed through ureteropyeloscopes are similarly long, small, and fragile and demand the greatest of care in handling and sterilization. These instruments can also be placed into long, flat, protective containers or coiled in padded protective boxes. They are often packaged for one-time use in a clear, semi-rigid plastic container (Fig. 12–4).

The processed instruments should be stored in an area with adequate space immediately adjacent to the endoscopic area. Although the arrangement of storage should be an individual decision, in general, similar instruments and those used together should be stored together for easy access. A key or map of the storage area should be available so that anyone working in the urologic department can gain immediate access to the desired instrument.

The exact container for the instrument will vary for the specific instrument and for the techniques used for either disinfection or sterilization. When gas sterilization is employed, a permeable tray must be used to allow total circulation of the gas. If the endoscopes are soaked in germicide for

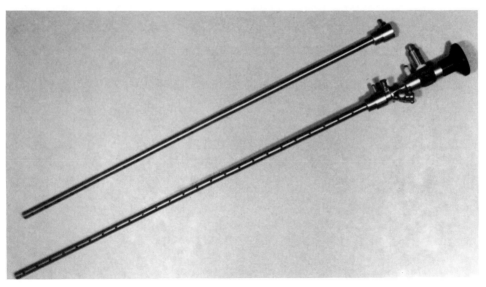

Figure 12–2. *The telescope is fit within a perforated sheath, which protects it from breakage and allows circulation of gas for sterilization.*

disinfection, then the tray itself is not subject to the process and instruments can be stored in other closed containers.

Instruments should be packaged to maintain sterility or cleanliness during storage. All instruments should be stored in covered, padded containers, and sterilized instruments should be wrapped to maintain this sterility. Coverings of plastic film provide the greatest protection after gas

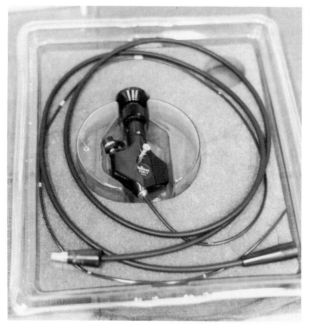

Figure 12–3. *A flexible ureteroscope is gently coiled on a bed of foam in its own tray for sterilization.*

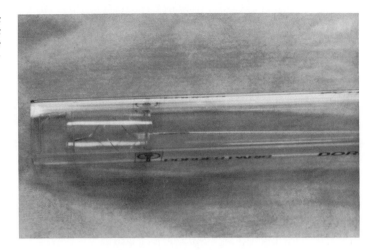

Figure 12–4. The ureteroscopic stone basket is within a clear plastic tube which protects the delicate wires but permits rapid visual identification.

sterilization (Fig. 12–5) However, a double-wrapping technique using paper or linen also provides a satisfactory covering to maintain sterility (Fig. 12–6).

Disinfection and Sterilization

Transmission of infectious disease between patients via endoscopes must be avoided by removing the causative organisms from the instruments or by rendering the organisms non-viable. The extent to which this must be achieved has been the subject of considerable controversy. Although the optimal situation would be to totally eradicate all organisms from instruments between uses, this is difficult to achieve because of the fragility of the instrument and its susceptibility to damage from the sterilization processes and difficult to define because of the nature of many infectious organisms.

It is difficult to define absolute death in a population of microorganisms. The life cycle of a contained population of microorganisms follows a growth

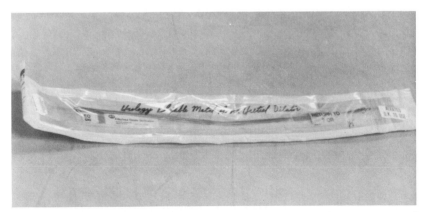

Figure 12–5. These ureteral dilators have been sterilized in a package consisting of paper on one side and clear plastic on the other.

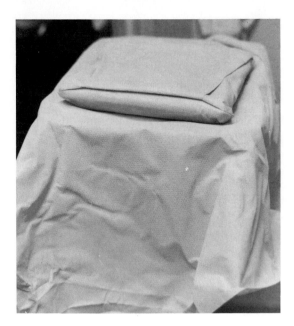

Figure 12–6. *The sterilized instrument is doubly wrapped in paper and is labeled on the outside for rapid identification.*

curve that includes an initial stationary or lag phase, a logarithmic or exponential growth phase, and a stationary phase during which the rates of multiplication and of death of the organisms are balanced. The population finally enters a death phase with a decline in population. Some populations of organisms, however, may survive for long periods of time even though the majority of organisms die early in an exponential fashion. One generally accepted criterion defining the death of a population of microorganisms is the inability of the organism to reproduce when placed in an optimal environment. Therefore, most tests evaluating processes for sterilization use a population of test organisms for which eradication can be determined. It is much more difficult to define the eradication of organisms that cannot be satisfactorily cultured or detected.

The techniques for processing instruments and ridding them of microorganisms are grouped according to their known effectiveness in eradicating specific populations of organisms. To provide assurance of the function of the process it is essential to employ techniques for checking this performance every time an instrument is cleaned and sterilized.

RISK CATEGORY

Three categories of medical and surgical instruments can be defined based on the seriousness of infection resulting from their use and the chance of infection. Spaulding and co-workers[4] describe these groups as critical, semi-critical, and non-critical.

Critical items carry a very high risk of inducing infection if they are contaminated by microorganisms. These items are passed directly into normally sterile areas of the body and should also be sterile. The *semi-critical group* includes equipment that comes into contact with intact epithelial surfaces but that does not ordinarily penetrate beyond the body's physical defenses. Endoscopes generally are classified in this group. The need for sterilization in this group remains the most controversial, and it has been considered that sterilization is desirable but not essential. Processing of these items should, at a minimum, destroy ordinary bacteria, tubercle bacilli, spores, and non-lipid viruses. Thorough mechanical cleaning, as noted previously, is the most important step. High level disinfection after mechanical cleaning has often been considered adequate for this group. *Non-critical items* either do not contact the patient or touch only unbroken skin. Sterility is not necessary for these items.

These categories are important in considering the degree of treatment needed for various levels of disinfection or for sterilization for any particular medical or surgical item. It would be ideal to provide sterility for all items if all processes used to achieve sterility were equally efficient, inexpensive, and rigorous to the instruments. However, this is not the case. In general, the severity of the process increases with the rate of treatment and with the effort expended to achieve sterility. Different materials within endoscopes can tolerate the cleansing processes to varying degrees, and some can be subjected only to the mildest processes with ingenuity.

DEFINITIONS

Sterilization has been defined as the destruction of all microbial life including highly resistant bacterial spores. Disinfection, in contrast, eliminates all recognized pathogenic bacteria and most other organisms, but not necessarily all organisms, including possible spores. Germicides are chemicals that have antimicrobial activity and can be used for disinfection. They usually kill ordinary vegetative forms of bacteria and can also be effective against tubercle bacilli, fungi, and non-lipid viruses. With prolonged contact, they may also be effective against spores. A disinfectant is a germicide used exclusively for killing microorganisms on non-living objects, whereas an antiseptic is a germicide used on skin or living tissue to inhibit or kill microorganisms.

Disinfection reduces the level of contamination by microorganisms but does not include the safety margin of overkill achieved with processes for sterilization. Disinfection has been categorized further into three levels: high, intermediate, and low.[4] High level disinfection can achieve chemical sterilization. By definition then it includes activity against spores, fungi, and viruses. Several disinfectants possess sporicidal activity, which has been considered an indication of high level disinfection. These include 2% glutaraldehyde, 8% formaldehyde solution, 70% alcohol, 6 to 10% stabilized hydrogen peroxide, and others that may be effective only with prolonged exposure.

Intermediate level disinfectants may not kill large numbers of bacterial spores but they must inactivate the tubercle bacillus. Some of these agents include 0.5% iodine, 70 to 90% ethanol, and isopropanol. Their effectiveness against viruses varies widely.

Low level disinfectants remove common vegetative bacteria but may be ineffective against tubercle bacilli, bacterial spores, or small non-lipid viruses. Activity can vary depending on the concentrations of bacteria and disinfectant and the length of exposure. Examples of low level disinfectants include quaternary ammonium compounds, mercurial compounds, and low concentrations of Iodophores and phenolic compounds.

The selection of the level of disinfection is related to the category of the surgical or medical item being treated. Critical items require sterilization, whereas non-critical equipment can be subjected to other levels of disinfection. The treatment of semi-critical items such as endoscopes remains most controversial. The tolerance of the instrument for sterilization must be considered as well as other practical factors such as the time needed for sterilization and the availability of alternative instrumentation.

Methods of Sterilization

As discussed previously, sterilization has been defined as the destruction of all life within the treated system. Various agents can achieve this; these agents may be either physical or chemical, including liquid, gaseous, and electromagnetic agents. However, severe conditions may be required in these processes to achieve death of the microorganisms. These severe conditions may also result in the destruction of the material being treated, depending on its fragility. Endoscopes are particularly fragile in this way because of the many different materials used in the construction of these instruments. Endoscopes cannot be exposed to wide variations in temperature, humidity, or chemical environment without the possibility of structural damage.

STERILIZATION BY HEAT

The standard agent for killing microorganisms has been heat. Dry heat requires high temperatures to achieve sterilization, and at reasonable temperatures is relatively slow. An open flame is routinely used to sterilize inoculating loops in the bacteriology laboratory, and immediate sterilization is thus achieved. At a temperature of 170°C (340°F) only 60 minutes' exposure may be required for sterilization, but as the temperature is reduced to 120°C (250°F), several hours' exposure is necessary. Dry heat has the advantage of being effective with all kinds of material including oils and closed containers that may not be permeable to humidity. However, it can be very destructive to many materials.

Moist heat is more rapidly effective under most conditions. Saturated steam at 120°C requires only a few minutes exposure to provide an extremely high probability of sterilization. Sterilization by steam under pressure is one of the most common techniques used clinically for sterilization and remains one of the least expensive. It can be employed for some of the urologic working instruments made entirely of metal such as biopsy forceps and metal sheaths but it must be avoided for equipment that can be damaged by heat and moisture, including essentially all endoscopes. Moist heat must be scrupulously avoided for endoscopic telescopes and for all flexible fiberoptic instruments.

STERILIZATION WITH ETHYLENE OXIDE

Ethylene oxide is a reactive molecule that alkylates nucleic acids, providing bacterial and sporicidal activity. Its effectiveness against spores has been related to the humidity within the system, with a maximum effect seen at 33 per cent. It has inactivated all viruses against which it has been tested.[3] Both temperature and exposure time as well as humidity are important and can be varied over standardized curves to provide sterilization of known microbial populations.

One of the major difficulties encountered with ethylene oxide has been the removal of the agent after an effective sterilizing cycle. Adherence of ethylene oxide to an instrument varies with the material composing the instrument, the packaging, and the parameters of the sterilizing cycle itself. Elution from flexible endoscopes may require several days at room temperature, while the same effect can be achieved within a few hours at higher temperatures. Newer sterilizers using high flows of gases have been successful in achieving rapid gas sterilization of endoscopes. Since ethylene oxide is a severe local irritant and has been implicated as a carcinogen, great care must be employed to ensure satisfactory aeration. Ethylene oxide can react with some epoxies used in fiberoptic flexible endoscopes. If instructions for sterilization are not available, then the manufacturer should be consulted prior to exposing instruments to ethylene oxide.

STERILIZATION WITH ULTRAVIOLET RADIATION

Ultraviolet radiation can alter DNA by cross-linking of adjacent residues and can be effective in killing microbial agents such as bacteria, yeast, and viruses. However, the ultraviolet light must penetrate the substance to sterilize, and thus with most instruments it has only a surface effect. Its application for sterilization of instruments is thereby severely limited. It has been used on a limited basis for maintaining sterility of instruments during storage.

STERILIZATION WITH GAMMA IRRADIATION

Gamma irradiation has been effective for sterilization, but because of the dangers associated with its use and the instruments required, it has been used mainly for bulk commercial applications. Although it has proved to be an economic and reliable sterilizing agent, it can irreversibly damage some materials in an as yet unpredictable way. It is not practical for use in general hospitals.

Sterilization Versus Disinfection of Ureteroscopes

There has been considerable controversy over whether to sterilize or disinfect endoscopes between uses. This controversy is not limited to urology but includes gynecology because of the use of laparoscopes and gastroenterology and general surgery because of the use of gastrointestinal endoscopes. With the increasing use of ureteroscopes and ureteropyeloscopes, the question of appropriate handling again arises.

Two strongly opposing camps hold different views in this controversy. One group supports sterilization and cites the risk of transmission of infectious disease between patients if the instrument is not fully sterilized even before use in each patient. This group cites the risks of transmission of otherwise undetectable diseases, such as non-A, non-B hepatitis and possibly AIDS. They further refer to the possibility of transmitting the "unknown."

On the other hand, there are those who consider that high level disinfection is satisfactory preparation before and after ureteroscopy. These workers cite the long-standing experience with disinfection in the preparation of urologic instruments and the voluminous evidence indicating its adequacy. For this group, the risk of transmitting spore-forming organisms or undetectable or unknown infectious diseases is nearly insignificant.

Overall, the recommendations put forth by the Centers for Disease Control appear reasonable. It is considered optimal to sterilize endoscopes before use but when this is not "feasible" high level disinfection constitutes adequate preparation.[2]

Care of Ureteropyeloscopes During Use

The fragility of ureteropyeloscopes must be considered in their handling throughout any procedure. As ureteropyeloscopes are set out for the procedure, a table with adequate surface area should be available to allow placement of the instruments without risk of other instruments lying upon them (Fig. 12–7). When a flexible ureteropyeloscope is used, ideally, it should be placed on a separate table to avoid the risk of a urethral sound or cystoscope landing on the delicate flexible tip.

In placing the instrument into the urethra and ureter, the urologist must keep in mind that the ureteroscope is long and narrow, and thus although a great deal of leverage can be generated with the instrument, the sheath and the telescope are relatively fragile and cannot withstand significant forces without bending or breaking. Immediately upon removal from the patient, blood and adherent material should be wiped from the surface of the instrument to prevent its drying and sticking to the surface and to maintain the instrument ready for repeated use.

At the completion of the procedure, the instrument should be removed from the operative field and carried to the processing area with specific individual care. Instruments should not be carried in groups and should not be carried with other heavy articles. Certainly the cost of several thousand dollars for replacing a flexible ureteropyeloscope justifies the effort necessary or for an individual to carry it alone to the processing area and follow through with its cleansing until it is placed into its padded, protective container.

Although ureteropyeloscopes are long, fine instruments that are among the most delicate endoscopes, with appropriate care and maintenance they can achieve a long, active use.

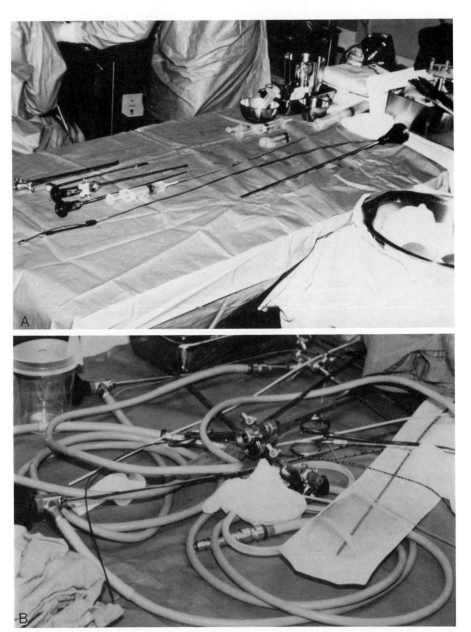

Figure 12–7. *The ideal operating room backtable separates the endoscopes (A) by size and purpose to maintain them ready for use and to free them of danger of damage. Overlying instruments and the "heaping" or "piling" effect (B) must be avoided.*

Availability of Endoscopes

Ureteroscopes should be stored in an area in the urologic suite where they can remain together and be readily identified for immediate access. Often a single instrument will not achieve the purpose during an endoscopic procedure and it will be necessary to use a second or third instrument, possibly along with the first. Although ideally every nurse and technician working in the urology suite should be familiar with the instruments, this is rarely achieved. Thus, it is worth an initial effort to establish an accessible storage system. A list of instruments and their locations should be available for anyone working within the suite. In our institution, we maintain instruments on shelves or in drawers with labels and have an index card system with cross-references indicating the specific shelf for each instrument. It is impossible to overemphasize that the endoscopes must be available and in working condition to be of any value to the urologist.

References

1. Bond WW, Favero MS, Mackel DC, and Mallison GF: Sterilization or disinfection of flexible fiberoptic endoscopes. AORN J 30:350, 1979.
2. Centers for Disease Control: Guidelines for the Prevention and Control of Nosocomial Infections. Atlanta, Centers for Disease Control, 1981.
3. Sidwell RW, Dixon GJ, Westbrook L, and Pulmodege EA: Procedure for the evaluation of the virucidal effectiveness of an ethylene oxide gas sterilizer. Appl Microbiol 17:790, 1969.
4. Spaulding EH, Cundy KR, and Turner FJ: Chemical disinfection of medical and surgical materials. In Lawrence CA and Block SS (eds.): *Disinfection, Sterilization and Preservation*. Philadelphia, Lea & Febiger, 1968, pp. 654–684.

Other Reading

Block SS (Ed.): *Disinfection, Sterilization and Preservation,* Ed. 3. Philadelphia, Lea & Febiger, 1983.

APPENDIX

Problem-Oriented Approach to the Hazards of Ureteropyeloscopy

R. ERNEST SOSA
JEFFRY L. HUFFMAN
DEMETRIUS H. BAGLEY

Hazards of Ureteropyeloscopy

The development of the ureteropyeloscope has helped the urologist gain access to the upper urinary tract for diagnostic and therapeutic purposes. While ureteropyeloscopy is an extension of endoscopic techniques used in the lower urinary tract, it is a far more demanding procedure with less room for error. The delicate nature of the ureter dictates gentle handling; therefore, in order to use these instruments safely and effectively, close attention to detail is imperative.

The focus of this section is on the problems most frequently encountered in the use of the ureteropyeloscope, beginning with possible pitfalls in patient preparation and including the entire process of ureteropyeloscopy.

Preparation for the Procedure

LACK OF FAMILIARITY WITH THE NATURE AND LOCATION OF THE PATIENT'S DISEASE

Identifying the ureteral or pelvic pathology, as well as potential "trouble spots" such as ureteral narrowing, displacement, or tortuosity, allows the urologist to estimate better the likelihood of success and also to prepare all the necessary ancillary equipment for performing the procedure. Pre-operative radiographs should permit the observation of the three-dimensional course of the ureter, with adequate visualization distal to an obstructing lesion. Therefore, a thorough radiologic evaluation undertaken prior to a ureteroscopic procedure should include excretory urography, retrograde pyelography, and if necessary computerized tomography (CT).

INADEQUATE OR IMPROPERLY FUNCTIONING INSTRUMENTS

Every instrument and piece of equipment that might possibly be needed to complete a procedure should be available and in good working order prior to beginning the procedure (see Chapter 4). Dilators, ureteropyeloscopes, stone baskets, an ultrasonic generator with probes, ureteral stents, and usually, a fluoroscopic unit are all required.

INSUFFICIENT OPERATING ROOM TIME ALLOWED FOR THE PROCEDURE

Ureteroscopic procedures require meticulous, coordinated work, which cannot be performed in a hurried manner. Ample time to work at a comfortable pace should be allowed, especially if stone manipulation is required.

Dilation of the Intramural Ureter

INABILITY TO FIND THE MEATUS

Mucosal edema, bladder trabeculations, marked hematuria, or an enlarged prostatic median lobe may hamper identification of the ureteral os. In these instances, indigo carmine may be administered intravenously. A flexible cystoscope may be used to see behind a large median lobe. If the meatus is still not visible, the procedure is terminated.

UNGUIDED METAL BOUGIE DILATOR WILL NOT ADVANCE ABOVE THE BLADDER HIATUS

If any resistance is encountered during the passage of the unguided bougies, do not apply more force; remove the dilator and use one of the methods of dilating over a guidewire (see Chapter 5).

INABILITY TO PASS A GUIDEWIRE INTO THE URETER

Under cystoscopic control, dilate the ureteral orifice with the unguided metal bougies, advancing them only as far as they pass easily. Then insert the ureteroscope to visualize the nature of the problem. Alternatively, use a small caliber ureteroscope that can pass into the undilated ureteral lumen. If it is possible to pass the guidewire under vision, remove the ureteroscope and proceed to dilate the tunnel as usual. If it is still not possible to pass the guidewire or to further advance the ureteroscope, abandon the procedure.

INADEQUATE DILATION OF THE TUNNEL

If upon inserting the ureteroscope it is noted that the intramural ureter has not been adequately dilated, remove the ureteroscope, re-introduce the cystoscope, and redilate the intramural ureter to size 15 F. When using balloon catheters, confirm the adequacy of dilation fluoroscopically.

URETERAL ORIFICE OR TUNNEL THAT RESISTS DILATION IN THE ABSENCE OF AN OBVIOUS ANOMALY

If an orifice or tunnel resists dilation, other types of dilators should be employed (metal bougies, graduated dilators, or balloon dilators). If dilation is still not possible, either pass a ureteral stent and attempt the procedure again in several weeks, or use an alternative method of treatment that does not require ureteroscopy.

FALSE PASSAGE OR PERFORATION OF THE URETERAL TUNNEL DURING DILATION

This complication is avoided by dilating the intramural ureter over a guidewire. However, if a perforation is identified after dilation, evaluate the damage with a ureteroscope. If the perforation is large, insert a ureteral stent and postpone the procedure for 4 to 6 weeks. If the ureteral damage is minimal, pass the ureteroscope into the true lumen and continue the procedure. Leave a ureteral catheter in place for 4 to 6 weeks.

Passage of the Ureteropyeloscope

URETEROSCOPE WILL NOT ENTER THE ORIFICE

If there is difficulty inserting the instrument into the orifice, first repeat the entire dilating process. Then align the ureteroscope with the three-dimensional course of the ureter and, with the beveled tip of the instrument rotated 180 degrees advance the ureteroscope toward the orifice. Rotation allows the upper lip of the os to be lifted by the bevel. Continue advancing the ureteroscope with the lumen within the field of vision. If a second guidewire can be placed, pass the ureteroscope over a wire.

UNABLE TO FIND THE URETERAL LUMEN

Do not attempt to advance the ureteroscope if the ureteral lumen is not in sight. Withdraw the instrument to an area in which the lumen is visible and then proceed slowly. Passage of a ureteral catheter or guidewire will often facilitate insertion of the instrument.

UNABLE TO ADVANCE THE URETEROSCOPE

Do not persist with insertion if the ureteroscope meets resistance. Tortuosity of the ureter can be overcome by advancing a 4-F ureteral catheter through the working channel beyond the ureteroscope, thus straightening the proximal ureter. If the ureter remains tortuous, persistent pressure will lead to ureteral perforation. In these instances of "fixed" tortuosity, the procedure may have to be terminated or a flexible ureteropyeloscope used. If a ureteral narrowing or a stricture prevents advancement of the ureteroscope, dilate the narrowed segment of ureter as described in Chapter 5.

POOR VISIBILITY

The advantages of direct visual access to the upper urinary tract are lost if endoscopic visibility is lost. This may occur because of bleeding or debris. Irrigation with a syringe through the side port of the ureteroscope or through a 4-F ureteral catheter helps to restore visibility. A blood clot may adhere to the telescope and obstruct visibility. Remove the telescope to check for clots if irrigation does not improve visibility. If visibility remains poor despite repeated irrigation, terminate the procedure.

AIR BUBBLES WITHIN THE URETER OR RENAL PELVIS

With the passage of instruments through the working channel, air is often introduced into the ureter. Air bubbles produce a significant restriction to visibility and should be removed by gentle aspiration with a small syringe through the side port of the ureteroscope or through a ureteral catheter. Alternatively, tilt the depressing table to move the bubbles to another position out of the visual field.

GOOD VISIBILITY, NO URETERAL NARROWING, BUT UNABLE TO ADVANCE THE URETEROSCOPE

Extrinsic pressure on the ureteroscope from a retroperitoneal tumor that decreases ureteral compliance, an overdeveloped psoas muscle, a large median prostatic lobe, or an erection can prevent advancement of the instrument. Further dilation of the ureter is unnecessary and unrewarding. Terminate the procedure and proceed with an alternative plan.

UNABLE TO PASS THE URETEROSCOPE INTO THE RENAL PELVIS BECAUSE OF RESPIRATORY EXCURSIONS

All patients are examined under general anesthesia with controlled respiration. The ureteroscope is advanced through the ureteropelvic junction under vision, during expiration. Alternatively, a 4-F ureteral catheter can be passed into the renal pelvis to fix the ureteropelvic junction in the "open" position.

URETERAL PERFORATION

A suspected ureteral perforation following a ureteroscopic procedure is identified or verified by injection of contrast material. As discussed previously, a self-retaining ureteral stent is left indwelling for 6 weeks, and the procedure is terminated.

PERFORATION OF THE RENAL PELVIS

When using the 70-degree lens, be aware that the tip of the telescope, in some models, may protrude outside of the ureteroscopic sheath. Therefore, advancing the instrument can result in perforation of the renal pelvis. The instrument should only be advanced with the 5-degree lens in place. With the 70-degree lens in place, the ureteroscope can be rotated to inspect the pyelocalyceal system, but it should not be advanced.

Stone Extraction

STONE MIGRATION

Position the patient with the shoulders slightly higher than the pelvis so as to create an uphill course for the distal ureter. Place the height of the irrigation fluid at a low level, maintaining flow at a minimum until the stone is engaged in the stone basket. Pass the stone basket by the stone gently, directing it, under vision, into an area where the stone is not adherent to the ureteral wall. Select beforehand a basket of appropriate size that is operational and in good repair. Do not permit others to view the stone or manipulate the ureteroscope until the stone is engaged in the basket.

UNABLE TO ENGAGE THE STONE IN THE BASKET

The most common reason for this difficulty is the use of an inappropriate stone basket. Even when the size of the basket is appropriate for the stone, the interstices between the wires may be too small to allow entry of the stone. Stone baskets with a greater number of wires (4 to 6), or with a spiral arrangement of the wires, have less room for embracing the stone than baskets of a similar size with fewer wires (4) arranged in a non-spiral pattern.

Another cause for difficulty in engaging a stone is that the stone is found in a capacious segment of ureter or in the renal pelvis. In the ureter, the passage of a ureteral catheter alongside the stone will often help trap the stone, facilitating its engagement in the basket. In the renal pelvis, tilting the cystoscopy table so that the stone comes to rest against the renal pelvis facilitates trapping the stone in the basket. Draining irrigant from the pelvis allows it to empty and forces the stone into the basket.

TRAUMATIZATION OF THE URETERAL WALL WITH THE STONE BASKET

The stone basket exits the ureteroscope sheath via the working channel at the six o'clock position. If the beak of the instrument is adjacent to edematous ureteral mucosa, the basket may perforate the mucosa and be advanced submucosally without being seen. Therefore, it is best to withdraw the ureteroscope slightly to an area that is more capacious, so that the tip of the basket can be seen as it enters the ureteral lumen. The basket should be passed beyond the stone without using force. If necessary, the ureteroscope can be carefully rotated until a "passage" where the stone is not adherent to the ureter is found. Advancement of the basket beyond the stone is monitored by fluoroscopy to ensure that the basket is in the ureter.

UNABLE TO EXTRACT AN OVERSIZED CALCULUS

Once the stone is engaged in the basket, the basket is closed. Ascertain that the ureteral mucosa has not also been trapped before the basket is closed. As the basket and stone are gently withdrawn down the ureter, continuous inspection of all points around the basket helps to ensure that the ureter is not trapped. Resistance to the removal of the stone in the basket suggests that the stone is too large to be safely brought down the ureter. Ultrasonic lithotripsy should be used to fragment the calculus, reducing it to a smaller, more easily removable size.

ULTRASONIC LITHOTRIPSY

Once the calculus is securely engaged in a stone basket, the sheath of the ureteroscope is snugged up to the basket so as to control the position of the stone. The telescope is removed, and the ultrasound probe is introduced under fluoroscopic guidance. Ultrasonic energy is delivered in 5- to 10-second bursts. Thermal injuries due to overheating of the ultrasonic probe are avoided by maintaining continuous irrigation during lithotripsy, with frequent palpation of the probe to detect excessive heat build-up before it can damage the ureter. Newer model ureteropyeloscopes with offset lenses allow the lithotripsy probe to be used under vision.

IMPACTED CALCULUS

If a stone is impacted in the ureter and cannot be engaged in a basket, then it is fragmented by ultrasonic lithotripsy directly (see Chapter 7). In these instances, if the offset ureteropyeloscope lens is not used, fluoroscopic control is mandatory.

RESIDUAL STONE FRAGMENTS

The urologist should attempt to remove all of the large stone fragments and as many of the smaller fragments as possible. This procedure often requires multiple trips up and down the ureter with the ureteroscope, resulting in mucosal trauma or bleeding with loss of optimal visibility. If all large fragments have been removed and only sandlike particles remain, a ureteral catheter may be left in place for 48 to 72 hours to maintain the ureteral lumen open and dilated until the mucosal edema subsides. The small stone fragments will pass. If larger fragments that are less likely to pass spontaneously cannot be removed, an indwelling ureteral stent is placed. The ureteroscopic procedure may be repeated at any time to remove the residual calculi.

UNABLE TO REMOVE THE CALCULUS

Stone removal from the upper urinary tract by ureteropyeloscopy may be unsuccessful 10 to 50 per cent of the time, depending on the location of the stone and other factors discussed in previous sections.

The physician and the patient should both be mentally prepared for alternative therapy, including open surgery, if ureteropyeloscopy is not successful. Stones inadvertently dislodged to the upper ureter or pelvis are often amenable to removal by percutaneous nephrostolithotomy or by ESWL.

Post-Operative Care

INFECTION

Infected urine is a contraindication to endoscopic manipulation of the upper urinary tract. Bacteria in an obstructed urinary system, or under the pressure of irrigation fluid, have access to the renal parenchyma from which systemic seeding can easily occur by pyelolymphatic and pyelovenous back-flow. Therefore, to prevent the potentially catastrophic complications of pyelonephritis and bacteremia, all patients must have cultures of their urine done pre-operatively. Infected urine should be sterilized with appropriate antibiotics prior to ureteroscopy. Any obstruction in the urinary system should be vented. It is recommended that all patients receive prophylactic intravenous antibiotics before they are taken to the operating room.

In the post-operative period, antibiotics are continued in accordance with the pre-operative urine culture findings, the procedure performed, and the presence of indwelling draining devices. A patient who has undergone a simple ureteroscopic procedure, whose urine is sterile, and in whom manipulation is minimal would receive oral antibiotics for only 24 to 48 hours after the procedure, whereas a patient with infected urine who was relieved of an obstructing stone may continue with intravenous antibiotics for several more days.

EXTRAVASATION-INDUCED HYPONATREMIA AND HEMOLYSIS

Extravasation of the irrigation fluid may occur as a result of ureteral trauma during ureteropyeloscopy. The nature of the irrigation fluid will determine the physiologic changes that occur when the extravasated fluid is absorbed into the vascular space and into the tissues. Normal saline will not produce changes in osmolality or electrolyte composition, but could place a patient with cardiac insufficiency into heart failure. Therapy requires the appropriate handling of the post-operative fluids and diuretics. If glycine is used as an irrigant, increased absorption will not result in a lower serum osmolality, but dilutional hyponatremia characterized by confusion, hypertension, and bradycardia can occur. Treatment is similar to that employed when the syndrome occurs following transurethral resection of the prostate. Water is potentially the most dangerous irrigant to use; increased absorption of water can cause a decrease in serum osmolality, producing hemolysis that could result in acute renal failure and death. Accordingly, the preferred irrigating solution for endoscopic intervention not requiring use of the electrocautery is normal saline. If cautery is required, glycine can be used.

PAIN

It is not uncommon for patients who have undergone ureteropyeloscopy to complain of mild pain in the lower abdominal quadrant corresponding to the side of the intervention. On palpation there is a mild degree of tenderness but rarely is rebound noted. This pain, which is thought to be due to dilation of the intramural ureter, usually dissipates over the next 24 hours.

Pain in the post-operative period may, however, herald more serious problems, particularly if it is accompanied by fever, peritoneal signs, or flank tenderness. If a draining ureteral catheter is not present, obstruction must be immediately ruled out. It is not unusual for mucosal edema following ureteral manipulation or a retained stone fragment to block a ureter if a stent has not been left in place. However, the presence of a catheter in the ureter is not a guarantee that there is no obstruction, since it is possible for debris, a clot, or a malpositioned catheter to prevent proper drainage. Once obstruction is diagnosed or strongly suspected, the system must be appropriately drained. The patient may experience transient colicky pain after removal of the catheter. Although this pain is usually of short duration, it may be severe enough to require the use of analgesics. It often appears to be the result of obstruction with a small blood clot, which usually passes within a few minutes to hours.

Pyelonephritis can be another potentially dangerous source of post-operative pain. Appropriate antibiotics determined by the results of urine cultures must be given intravenously, and obstruction must be ruled out as discussed previously.

A retroperitoneal collection of fluid from extravasation or bleeding could also produce ureteral obstruction or peritoneal irritation and therefore pain and fever. If extravasation is documented, then the ureter should be catheterized to divert the urine during healing of the injury. If a hematoma is suspected, the patient's hematocrit should be checked frequently to help determine if watchful waiting or intervention is needed for resolution of the problem.

Pain may also appear in any area of the body as a result of pressure injury from lack of adequate padding of the body during the procedure. Treatment in such cases is symptomatic.

FOLLOW-UP

Urine cultures should be repeated in the post-operative period regardless of the status of the pre-operative cultures. In a hospital environment, it is not unusual to acquire a new infection following endoscopic manipulation, or a new infecting organism may be selected by antibiotic therapy and cause symptoms. Treatment is then dictated by the results of the sensitivity tests of the bacteria.

Following ureteroscopic procedures, appropriate radiologic studies should be performed in all patients to ascertain the integrity of the urinary tract. After a short, routine case an excretory urogram may be performed at a post-operative visit 6 weeks following the procedure. More complicated cases that require post-operative indwelling ureteral catheters may be studied by retrograde pyelography at the time the catheter is removed, with an excretory study performed at a later date.

Index

Page numbers in *italics* indicate illustrations; page numbers followed by the letter t indicate tables.